IMAGES
of America

CHICAGO'S NURSE PARADE

About the Authors

Carolyn Hope Smeltzer, Frances R. Vlasses, and Connie R. Robinson are nurses. They were not nurses during the era of the Chicago Nurses Day Parade, but they have gone to schools and/or worked at many of the hospitals that participated, and have great respect for the nurses who created this visible history for us to relive.

Carolyn is a partner in PricewaterhouseCoopers' healthcare advisory practice. She serves as a trustee on several healthcare boards including Advocate Healthcare System and Sisters of Charity of Leavenworth Health System. She is on the President's Board of Regents of Loyola University, Chicago. She lives, golfs, and swims in both Chicago and Lake Geneva, Wisconsin. *Lake Geneva in Vintage Postcards*, her second book for Arcadia, written with coauthor Martha Kieffer Cucco, will be published in 2005.

Fran is a faculty member at Loyola University, Niehoff School of Nursing. She is a volunteer puppy raiser for Canine Companions for Independence, raising assistance dogs for people with disabilities.

Connie is a Clinical Nurse Associate in Pediatric Nephrology at the University of Chicago Children's Hospital. She is actively involved in several organizations that raise the public's awareness of the need for organ donations. She and her son Patrick reside in the historic Hyde Park neighborhood of Chicago.

Carolyn and Fran coauthored the book *Ordinary People, Extraordinary Lives: The Stories of Nurses* (Sigma Theta Tau International Publishers, 2003). This coffee table book highlights the often silent stories of how nurses lead their lives, caring for patients, community, family, and friends. Connie, Fran, and Carolyn are committed to uncovering nurses' stories and preserving the history of both nursing and Chicago.

Notes from the Authors

"Of course you both know of the Nurses Day Parade. . . ." Fran and Carolyn were puzzled by Father Paul Novak's comment. After being educated as nurses, living in Chicago, and listening to virtually hundreds of nursing stories when coauthoring the book *Ordinary People, Extraordinary Lives: The Stories of Nurses*, how could we have missed a ten-year-long event about nursing? This began a journey of questions and surprises.

Father Paul Novak, seeing our surprise, put us in touch with Father Conrad at Our Lady of Sorrows Basilica who became our guide. We were soon joined by Janet Boivin, who brought the tools to search for testimony from participants and who published the first story about the Nurses Day Parade in 45 years in *Nursing Spectrum* (2004).

Connie Robinson's ingenuity completed the team. Each of us recognized the importance of sharing this historic finding. Yet, despite the fact that all four of us talked to colleagues and acquaintances throughout the country for over a year, it became evident that the world's "shortest parade" was also Chicago's best-kept secret.

As so often happens with storytelling, what started as a simple retelling of a tale about Carolyn's mother, a Chicago nurse, during a reflection at Old St. Patrick's Church on Mother's Day, 2003, led us once again to a deeper appreciation of our heritage. Now we invite you to discover the Nurses Parade, a parade that gave nurses their "day of glory" in a city that Colonel John "Jack" Reilly appropriately called "the Parade Capital of the World."

IMAGES
of America

CHICAGO'S NURSE PARADE

Carolyn Hope Smeltzer with
Frances R. Vlasses and Connie R. Robinson

ARCADIA
PUBLISHING

ISBN 978-1-5316-1923-7

Published by Arcadia Publishing
Charleston, South Carolina

Library of Congress Catalog Card Number: 2004114586

For all general information contact Arcadia Publishing at:
Telephone 843-853-2070
Fax 843-853-0044
E-mail sales@arcadiapublishing.com
For customer service and orders:
Toll-Free 1-888-313-2665

Visit us on the Internet at www.arcadiapublishing.com

Dedication:

To the nurses who came before us, creating a heritage of caring, and to those now and in the future who safeguard this legacy.

In memory of Dr. Julia A. Lane, Dean, Niehoff School of Nursing, Loyola University Chicago, 1971–1991.

CONTENTS

ACKNOWLEDGMENTS

The late Father Clarence M. Brissette, O.S.M., the national director of the *Sorrowful Mother Novena* at Our Lady of Sorrows Basilica was the founder and driving force behind the parade. His writings in the *Novena's* weekly newsletter reveal his great respect and passion for the nursing profession.

Father Paul Novak, assistant provincial of the Religious Order of Servants of Mary (Servites), appreciated storytelling and serendipitously shared the story of the Chicago Nurses Day Parade with us. Without his directions and belief in us, perhaps the contents of *Chicago's Nurse Parade* would still lay silent in the archives. He directed us to Father Conrad and to the archives of Our Lady of Sorrows Basilica to uncover the story of the parade.

Father Conrad Borntrager, religious order of the Servants of Mary (Servites), provincial archivist at Our Lady of Sorrows Basilica, meticulously preserved the history of the parade. Father Conrad also marched in several of the parades as a member of the St. Philip High School band. Father Conrad was welcoming and supportive in resurrecting the memories of the parade. He enthusiastically opened up the parade files for the first time in over 40 years and provided guidance and editing of this book. He was gracious in letting us share the parade's photography and memorabilia with the rest of the world.

Janet Boivin, R.N., editorial director of the greater-Chicago, tri-state *Nursing Spectrum*, immediately saw the value in learning more about the parade and its participants. Janet highlighted the parade in the November 2003 issue of *Nursing Spectrum*, requesting testimony from those who marched in or remembered the parade. Janet shared these pictures and sentiments of the parade by authoring "Chicago Nurses' Parade," for *Nursing Spectrum* in January, 2004.

Dr. Sheila Haas, Dean, and Dr. Ida Androwich, Professor, Niehoff School of Nursing, Loyola University Chicago, fostered an environment where faculty, alumni, and students work, think, learn, teach, create, and author together.

Samantha Gleisten, acquisitions editor for Arcadia Publishing, believed that stories about nurses, parades, and Chicago would be of interest to all. She fully understood that stories about all three would be a powerful and worthy publication.

ARCHDIOCESE OF CHICAGO

Office of the Archbishop

Post Office Box 1979
Chicago, Illinois 60690-1979

A COMMENDATION

The authors of this book have done a favor to the Archdiocese and the city of Chicago in rescuing this piece of history and bringing it to public notice. Though the Chicago Nurse Parade continued for no more than a decade, it succeeded "in placing nursing on a national pedestal".

The memory of that Parade, brought to us in this text and in an abundance of photographs, re-focuses attention on the nursing profession and stirs our gratitude anew.

The contribution of the Catholic Church is integral to the story of the Parade. My prayer is that this tradition of expert and deeply humane care of the sick and the dying may continue to draw direction and strength from faith in Christ and a Catholic way of life.

Francis Cardinal George, O.M.I.
Archbishop of Chicago

OFFICE OF THE MAYOR

CITY OF CHICAGO

RICHARD M. DALEY
MAYOR

Chicago's Nurse Parade celebrated nursing in our city for the ten years from 1949 to 1958. Supported by government and community leaders throughout the city and organized by Clarence M. Brissette, O.S.M., director of Sorrowful Mother Novena, the Parade was a way to honor our city's nurses as well as help recruit more men and women into the nursing profession. The first Nurse Parade was modest, with only two floats and four bands. But by the tenth anniversary of the Parade, there were 4,000 marching uniformed nurses, over 30 bands and 100 floats from hospitals and nursing schools throughout the city.

I commend the authors of this book, Carolyn Smeltzer, Frances R. Vlasses and Connie Robinson for their work to highlight this important part of Chicago's history, as well as Father Conrad Borntrager of the religious order of the Servants of Mary (Servites), provincial archivist at Our lady of Sorrows Basilica, who preserved the history of the parade for future generations to enjoy.

Richard M Daley

The Honorable Richard M. Daley
Mayor, City of Chicago
November 4, 2004

INTRODUCTION

Chicago's Nurses Day Parade is considered the only consecutive "one of a kind nurses' parade" in the nation, yet remains relatively unknown. This book revisits the history of the nurses' parade in the "City of Parades," Chicago. Read, view, and feel the pride of nurses marching, the enthusiasm of spectators cheering as they lined the streets of Jackson Boulevard, the beauty of the floats gliding by, the sounds of the bands playing, and the impressive number of parade supporters honoring nurses.

This book illustrates the planning efforts, budget, floats, media coverage, dignitary participation, and pronouncements of the parade and ceremonies to help nurses gain visibility. The beautiful photography provides chronological images that may cause you to reflect on the nurses that went before us. Your mind and imagination may wonder . . . if the dates of the parade were not noted and the photography did not highlight the dress and style of the 1950s, could this be a book about today's nurses?

It is our hope that after reading this book and seeing all the magnificent images from the decade of the Chicago Nurses Day Parade that you will have a renewed sense of respect and pride for nurses, who each day forego fame and fortune to care for the ill and injured members of our society. This book provides an opportunity to learn from nursing's past and appreciate and respect historic nursing moments and memories. It also provides a powerful example of community, merchants, media, church, and government all working together to help nurses gain visibility and address the nurse shortage.

We now invite you to read, visualize, and feel the excitement, support, respect, caring, and honor that surrounded the Nurses Day Parade in Chicago. Experience the parade giving nurses their "day of glory."

One

Let The Word Go Forth
Nurses Day Proclamation

Clarence M. Brissette, O.S.M., inspired the development of "the World's Largest, Shortest Parade" from its inception in 1948 to the final parade in 1958. He stated that the parade's purpose was to place "a noble profession on a national pedestal where it rightly belongs" (*New World*, June 15th, 1949). Father Brissette had the first Nurses Day declared by Mayor Kennelly and Governor Stevenson in 1949. Thereafter, until 1958, each Chicago mayor and governor of Illinois proclaimed Nurses' Day. By 1958 the parade was viewed by 100,000 spectators and included 100 hospital floats and 4,000 nurse participants. The parade received support from city, state, community, merchants, and national public figures as well as from radio, television, and newspapers. The parade was featured in every Chicago newspaper as well as some national newspapers. The 1957 Chicago Nurses Day Parade was filmed by three crew members from Ardex Film of Wichita, Kansas. They were developing a nurse vocational movie to be distributed worldwide.

The parade evolved from a Friday night pilgrimage organized and led by Father Brissette. Starting with the first parade in 1949 and continuing through its history, pilgrimages were common, and Catholic prayers to the Virgin Mary were publicly recited by nurses and supporters.

Father Brissette believed a good nurse had more influence at the bedside than a minister, priest, or rabbi. He said that since the average pay of the nurses had not kept pace with modern wages, the motives in wanting to be a nurse spring from something higher than material compensation, such as the fulfillment of a calling or longing of the soul: "How can I be of assistance to others?" He believed the nursing profession was a product of Christianity founded on the principle of love and giving of self. He believed the nursing profession appealed to those who are good and noble.

"When we speak to people who have been or are patients in a hospital and when they praise the attending nurse it is most always in these terms: 'so kind, so patient, so understanding.' They seldom talk of the nurse in terms of efficiency, how dexterous they handle the hypodermic needle, take a blood test or temperature. . . . Nurses are appreciated and remembered mostly in terms of kindness." (Clarence Brissette, *Novena Notes*, May 18, 1956, 3.)

Although the *Novena Notes* newsletters unabashedly linked images of nursing with religion and the Virgin Mary, Father Brissette, in his own words, said the parade was non-denominational and all, regardless of creed or religion, were invited and welcomed to participate. At the end of the parade, nurses and others entered a candlelit Basilica for services and prayers. Nurses could renew their "Nurses Pledge" and light a candle. This was a striking, powerful, emotional, solemn, and dramatic scene as all could feel the presence of nursing.

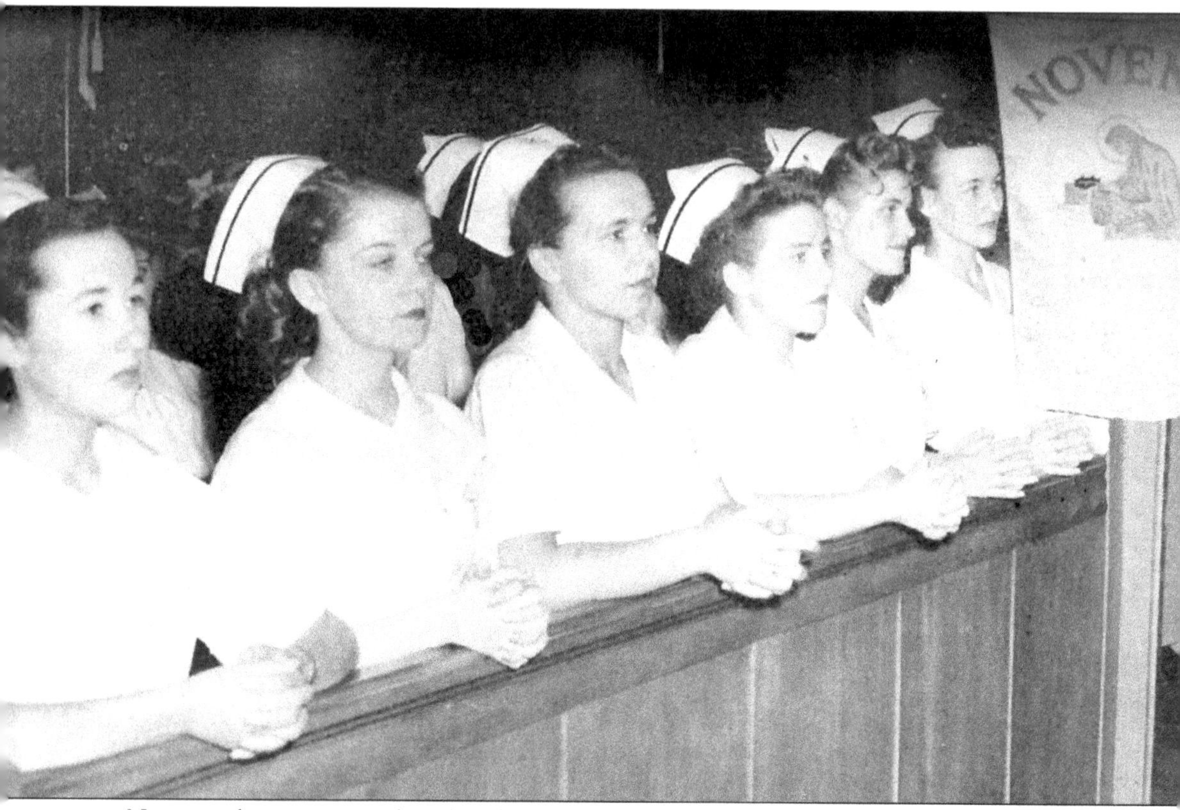

Nurses and supporters gathered at the National Shrine on July 16, 1948, to pay homage to St. Camillus de Lellis, the patron saint of hospitals and the sick. This was a prelude to the first Nurses Day Parade, held in 1949. (*Novena Notes*, August 6, 1948, cover.)

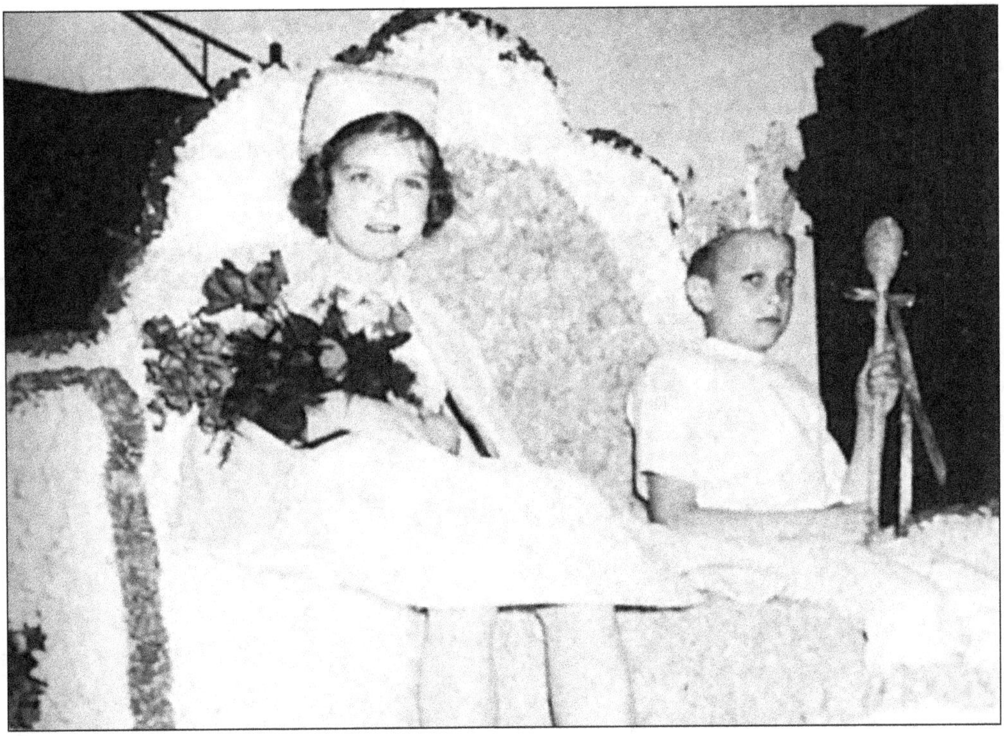

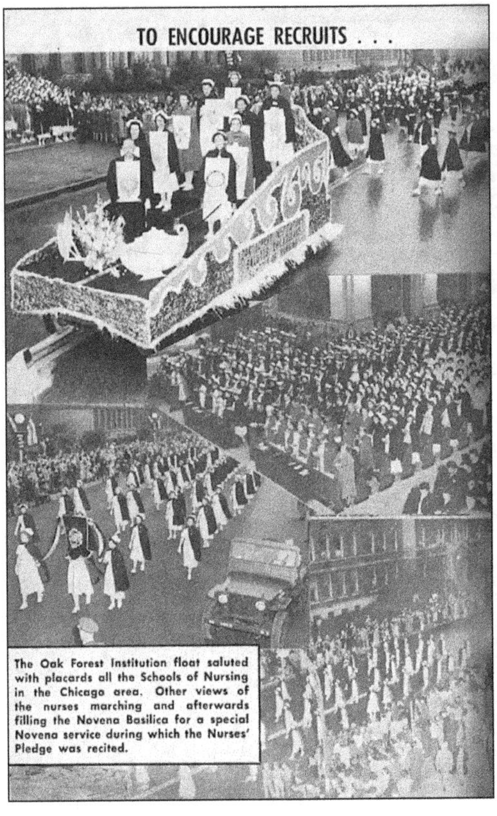

TO ENCOURAGE RECRUITS . . .

The Oak Forest Institution float saluted with placards all the Schools of Nursing in the Chicago area. Other views of the nurses marching and afterwards filling the Novena Basilica for a special Novena service during which the Nurses' Pledge was recited.

Teachers asked, "Father, why so much concern about nurses, why the annual parade to glorify nurses . . . why not give school teachers the same break?" Father Brisette's response was, "We agree heartily something should be done for the teaching profession . . . but nurses are teachers too." (*Novena Notes*, May 18, 1956, 8.)

Recruiting nurses into the profession was a focus of the Nurses Day Parades. "The nursing profession is most exacting in its demands and neither desire for gain nor fame are sufficient to draw young people within its ranks. It appeals to the dedicated, those consumed with a desire to help their fellow men." (*Novena Notes*, May 9, 1958, 9.)

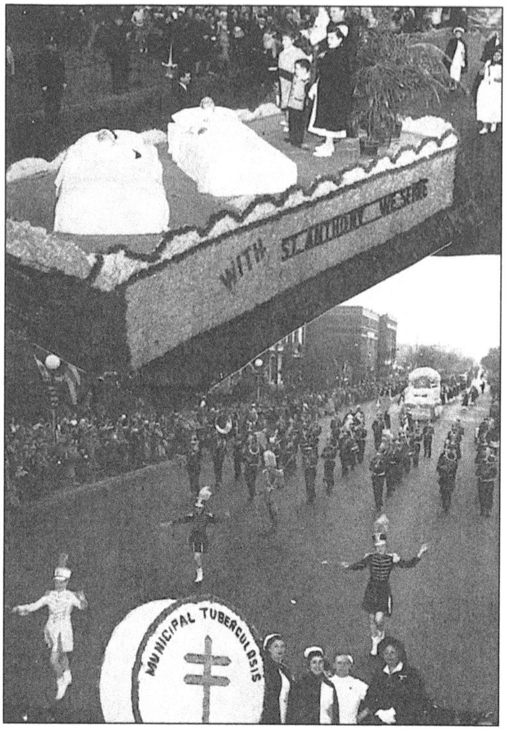

Mr. Sachs, city treasurer, represented the city at the parade in Mayor Daley's absence. Mr. Sachs stated, "I am on the Governor's Welfare Board so I know the critical need of more nurses in hospitals and institutions to say nothing of the deplorable shortage existing in private practice. I believe the city and state should do everything possible to encourage young people to go into the nursing field and at the same time everything practical should be done to make the pay and working conditions of the nurse more attractive." (*Novena Notes*, June 10, 1955, 10.)

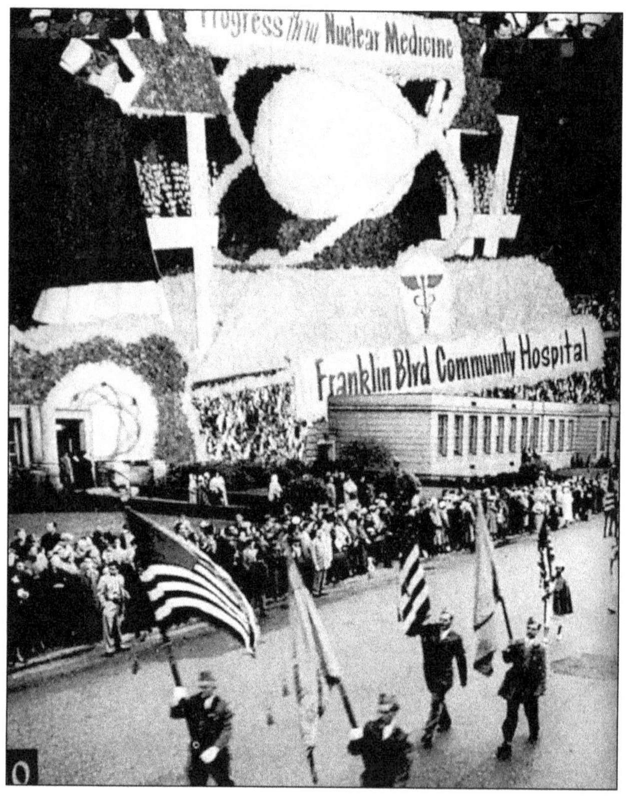

"Although the Nurses Day Parade was sponsored by the Sorrowful Mother Novena, it was nonsectarian and non-denominational. All were invited to participate regardless of race, color or creed." (*Novena Notes*, May 30, 1958, 10.)

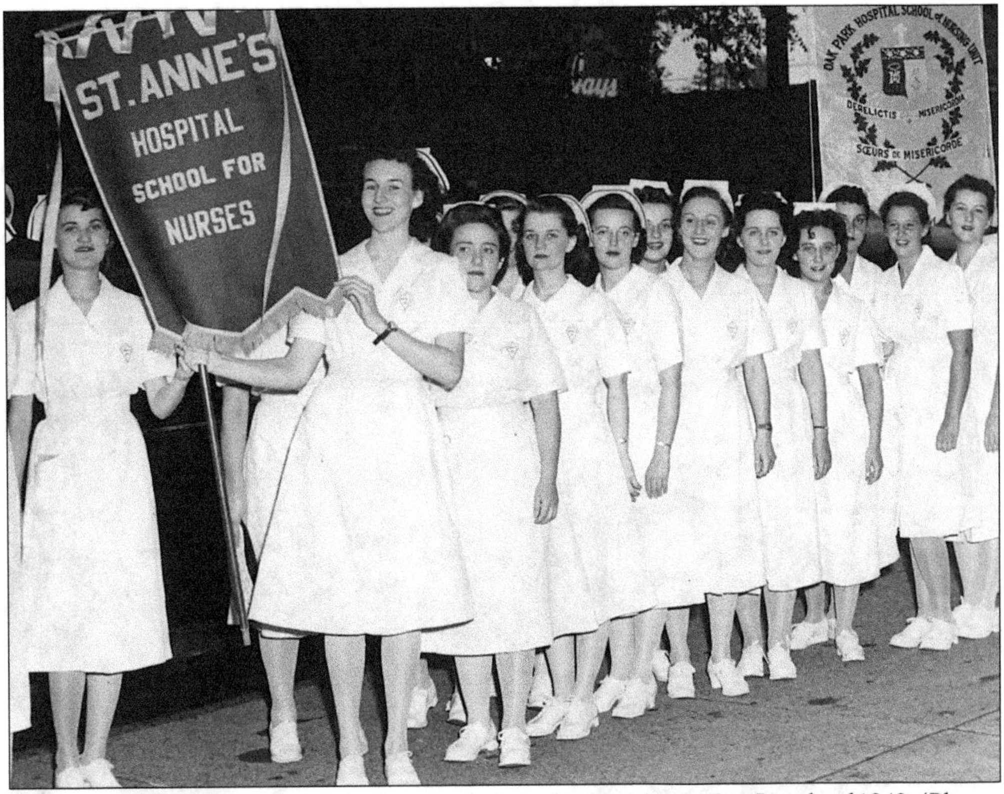

St. Anne's nurses, in 1948, marched in a prelude to the first Nurses Day Parade of 1949. (Photos also appear in *Novena Notes*, August 6, 1948, 8.)

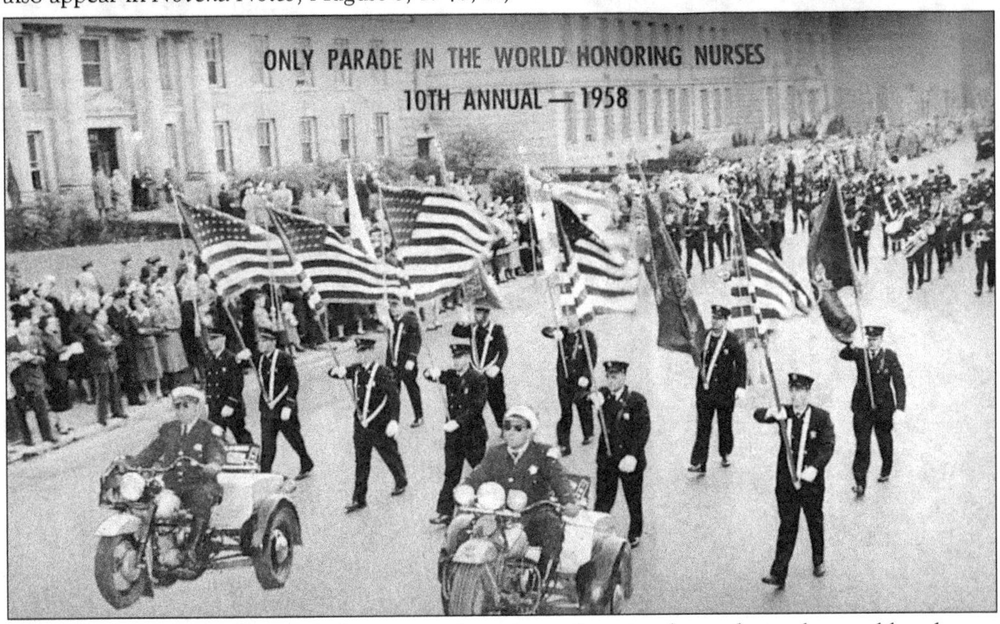

The Chicago Nurses Day Parade was cited as the only annual parade in the world to honor nurses consecutively for a decade. The tenth parade, held in 1958, was spectacular. (*Novena Notes*, May 30, 1958, cover.)

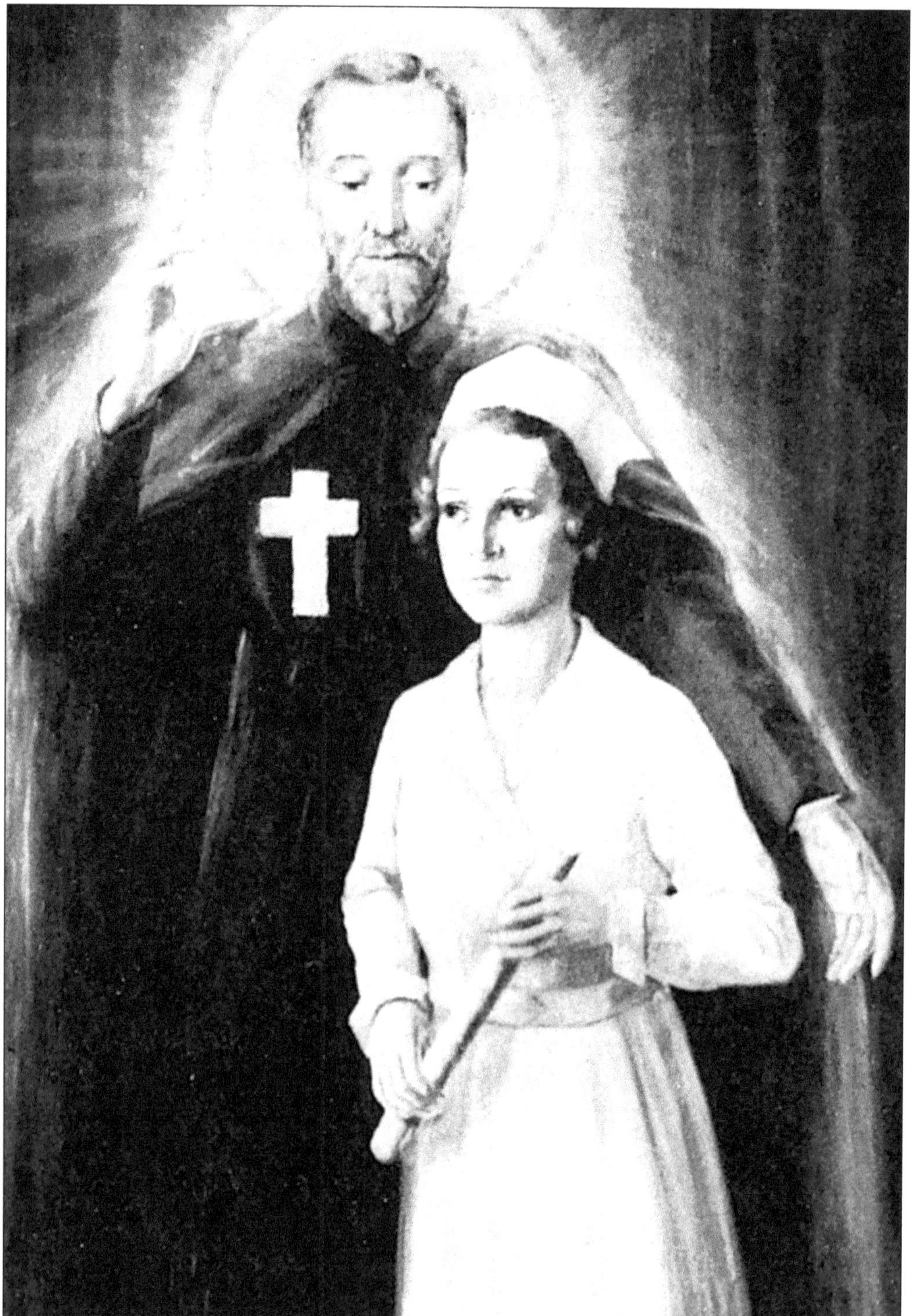

St. Camillus' story is dramatic and colorful. Before he turned to religion he was a confirmed gambler and soldier of fortune. Uninterrupted suffering marked his life for 46 years. This *Novena Notes* cover is in honor of him and of nurses. (*Novena Notes*, July 15, 1949, cover.)

Chicago's mayor proclaimed September 15, 1950, as Nurses Day in Chicago and as the date for the second official Nurses Day Parade. (*Novena Notes*, Sept. 8, 1950, 9.)

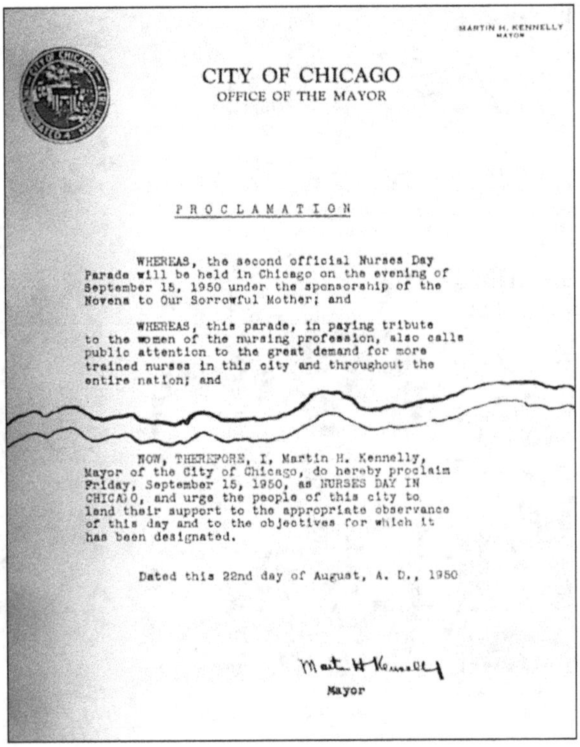

MARTIN H. KENNELLY
MAYOR

CITY OF CHICAGO
OFFICE OF THE MAYOR

PROCLAMATION

WHEREAS, the second official Nurses Day Parade will be held in Chicago on the evening of September 15, 1950 under the sponsorship of the Novena to Our Sorrowful Mother; and

WHEREAS, this parade, in paying tribute to the women of the nursing profession, also calls public attention to the great demand for more trained nurses in this city and throughout the entire nation; and

NOW, THEREFORE, I, Martin H. Kennelly, Mayor of the City of Chicago, do hereby proclaim Friday, September 15, 1950, as NURSES DAY IN CHICAGO, and urge the people of this city to lend their support to the appropriate observance of this day and to the objectives for which it has been designated.

Dated this 22nd day of August, A. D., 1950

Martin H Kennelly
Mayor

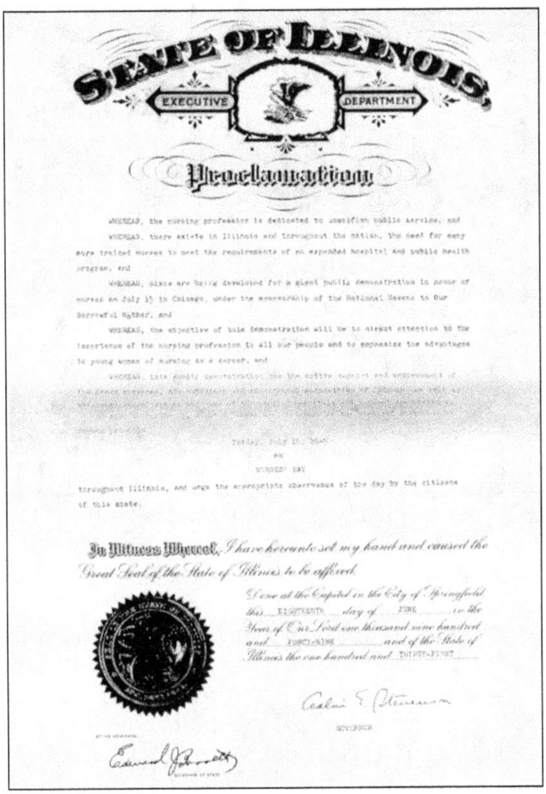

STATE OF ILLINOIS,
EXECUTIVE DEPARTMENT

Proclamation

In Witness Whereof, I have hereunto set my hand and caused the Great Seal of the State of Illinois to be affixed.

Illinois Governor Adlai Stevenson signed the proclamation for Nurses Day in 1949. (*Novena Notes*, July 8, 1949, 8.)

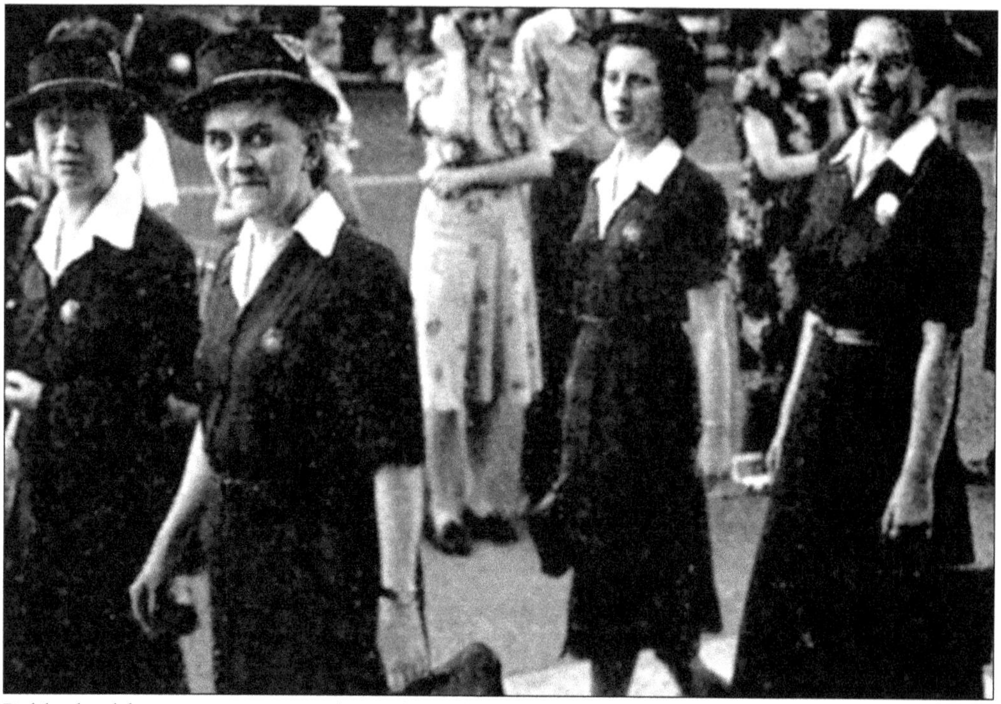

Public health nurses are pictured marching. (*Novena Notes*, August 6, 1948, 9.)

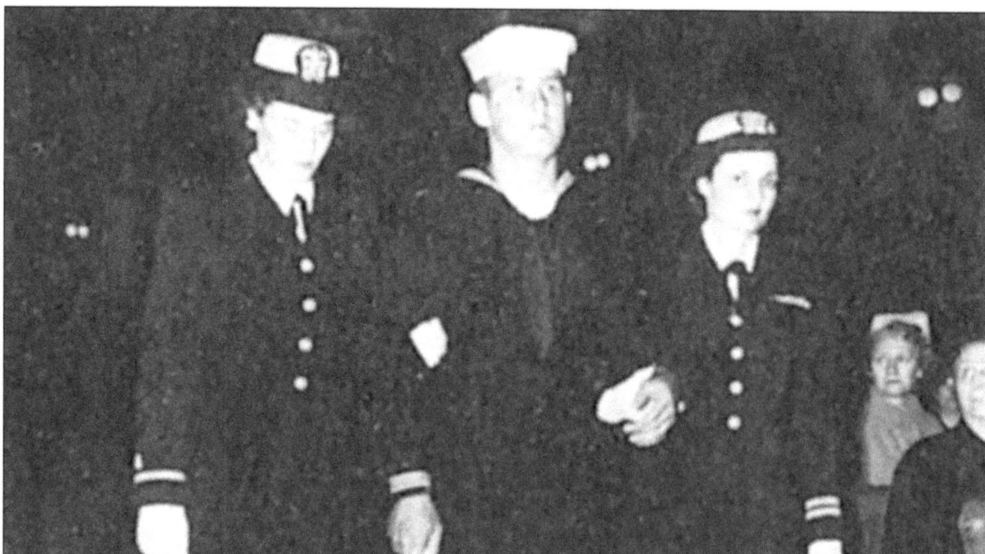

"A girl who enters the nursing profession must be fundamentally unselfish; she must be able to smother her own will to serve others. Nursing is a vocation in which one voluntarily takes on suffering that others might suffer less. A Christian nurse adds nobility to the care of the sick with the concepts of sharing in Christ's work of healing bodies which are God's temples. Nurses live in God's grace, are like priests . . . bearers of God's gift to humanity. . . . Tonight the Sorrowful Mother Novena salutes the nursing profession . . . praying each week that the Mother of God will inspire other noble women to serve as God's hands in ministering to the world," wrote Stephen M. Gibbons, O.S.M., assistant Novena director. (*Novena Notes*, May 22, 1953, 8.)

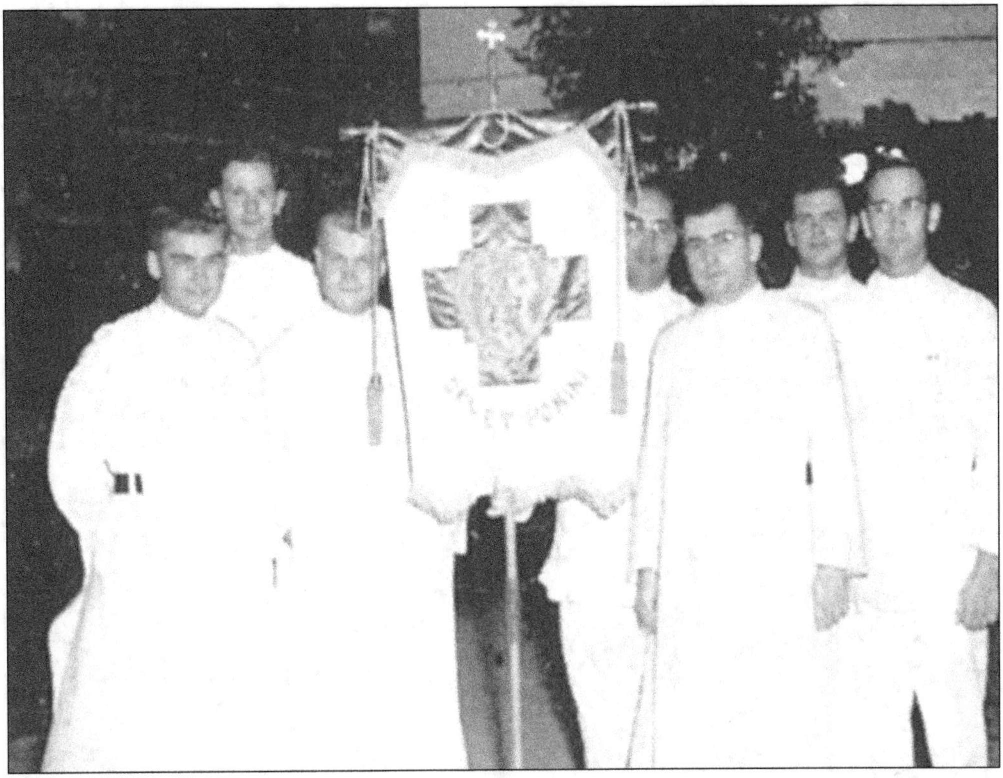

Alexian Brothers Hospital's male nurses carry a banner with a large insignia of a cross. St. Camillus created the "Red Cross" symbol that is now used by the International Red Cross Organization. (*Novena Notes*, August 6, 1948, 9.)

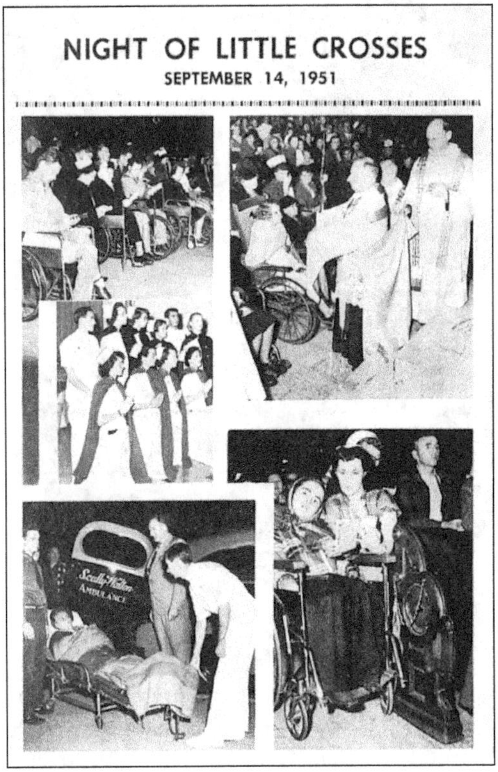

NIGHT OF LITTLE CROSSES

SEPTEMBER 14, 1951

Nurses also participated in the Night of the Little Crosses, which also gave visibility to the work of nurses. (*Novena Notes*, October 5, 1951, back cover.)

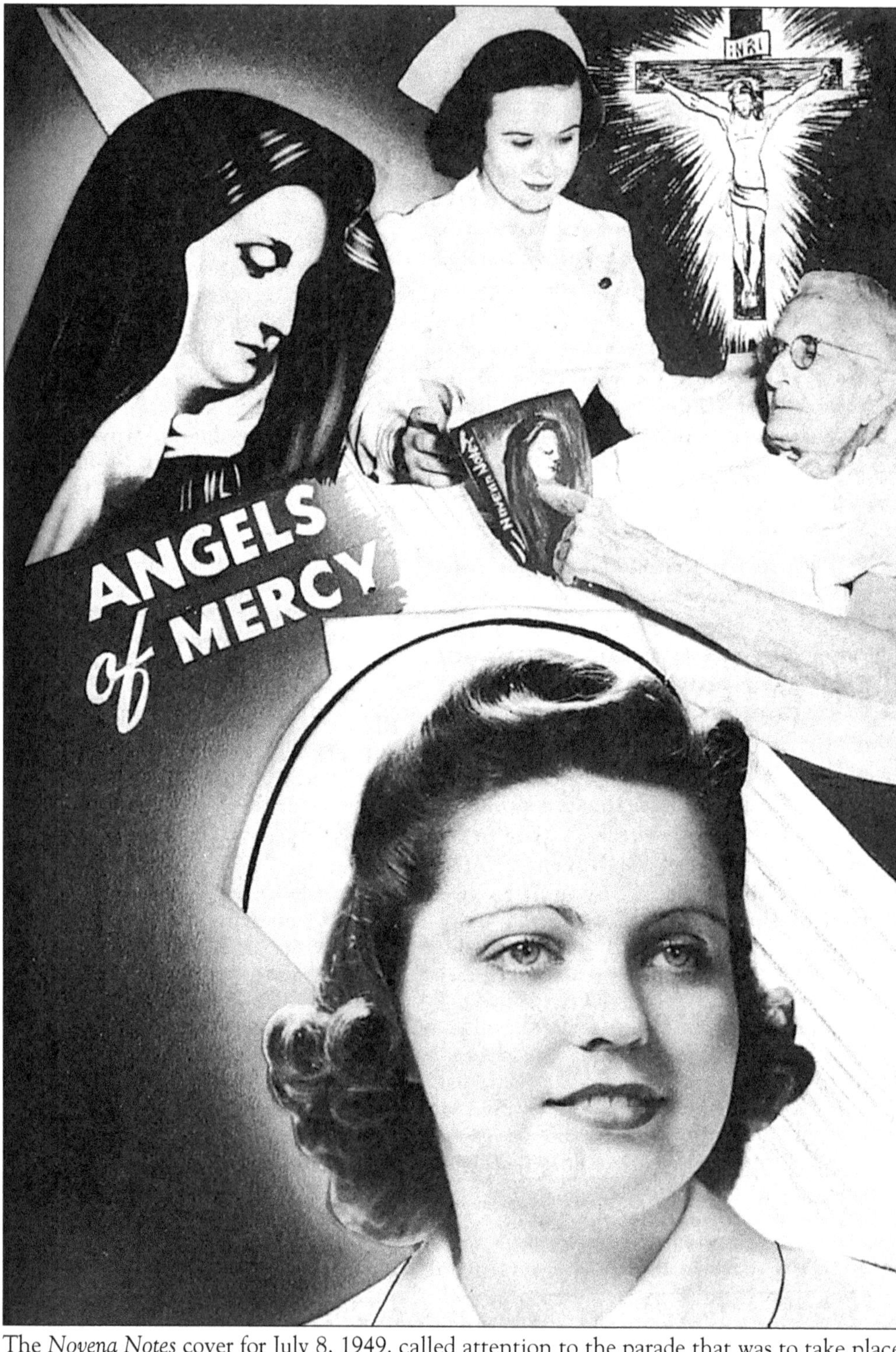

The *Novena Notes* cover for July 8, 1949, called attention to the parade that was to take place on July 15, 1949, at 7 p.m. The parade was to honor St. Camillus, universal patron of nurses and hospitals. (*Novena Notes*, July 8, 1949, cover.)

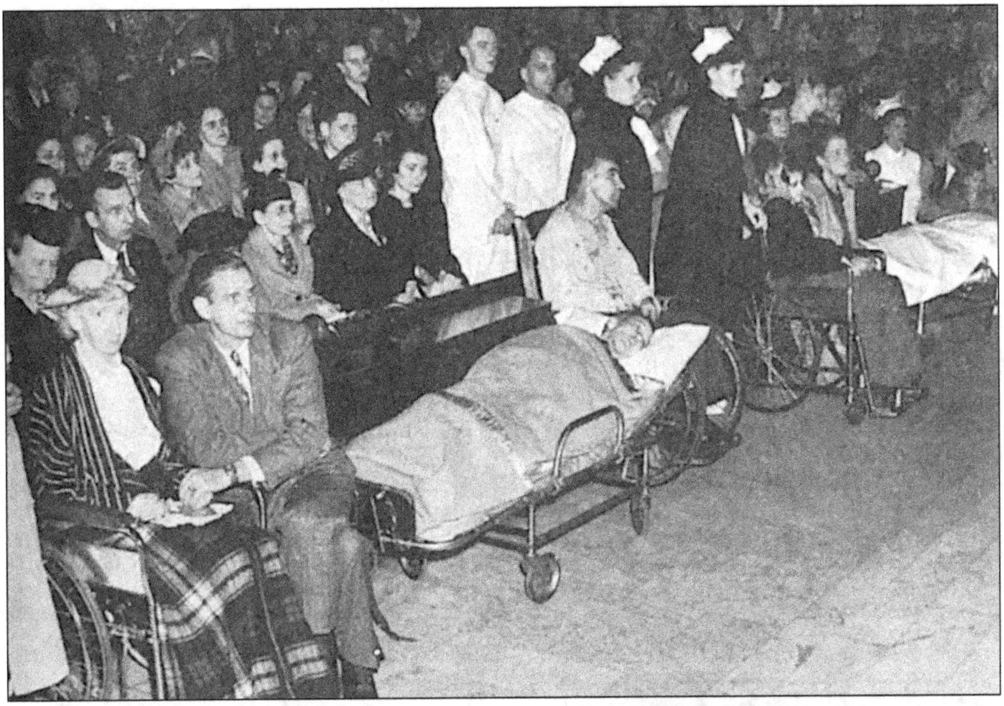

Many sick or disabled individuals were brought into Our Lady of Sorrows Basilica on stretchers, in wheelchairs, and in hospital beds during the "sick and shut-in night." Nurses were ready and willing to care for the participants. The "sick and shut-in night" provided visibility to the nurses' work, similar to the visibility brought by the parade. (*Novena Notes*, Sept. 8, 1950, cover.)

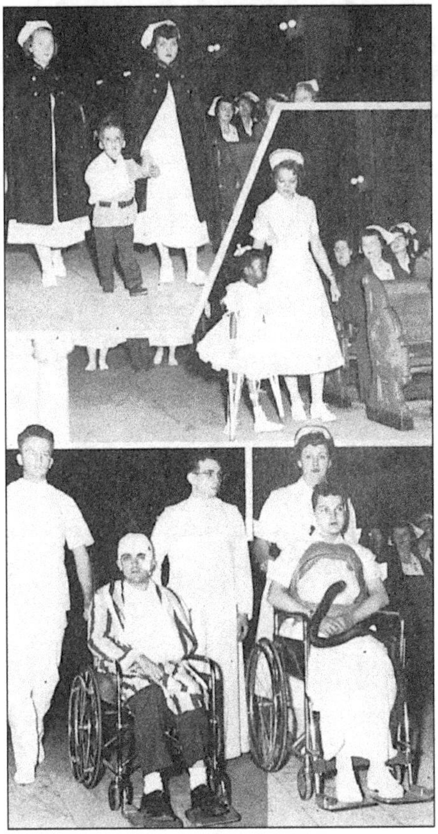

Nurses brought the sick to the church for a special service for the "sick and shut-ins." The nurses also provided care during the service. (*Novena Notes*, June 12, 1953, 9.)

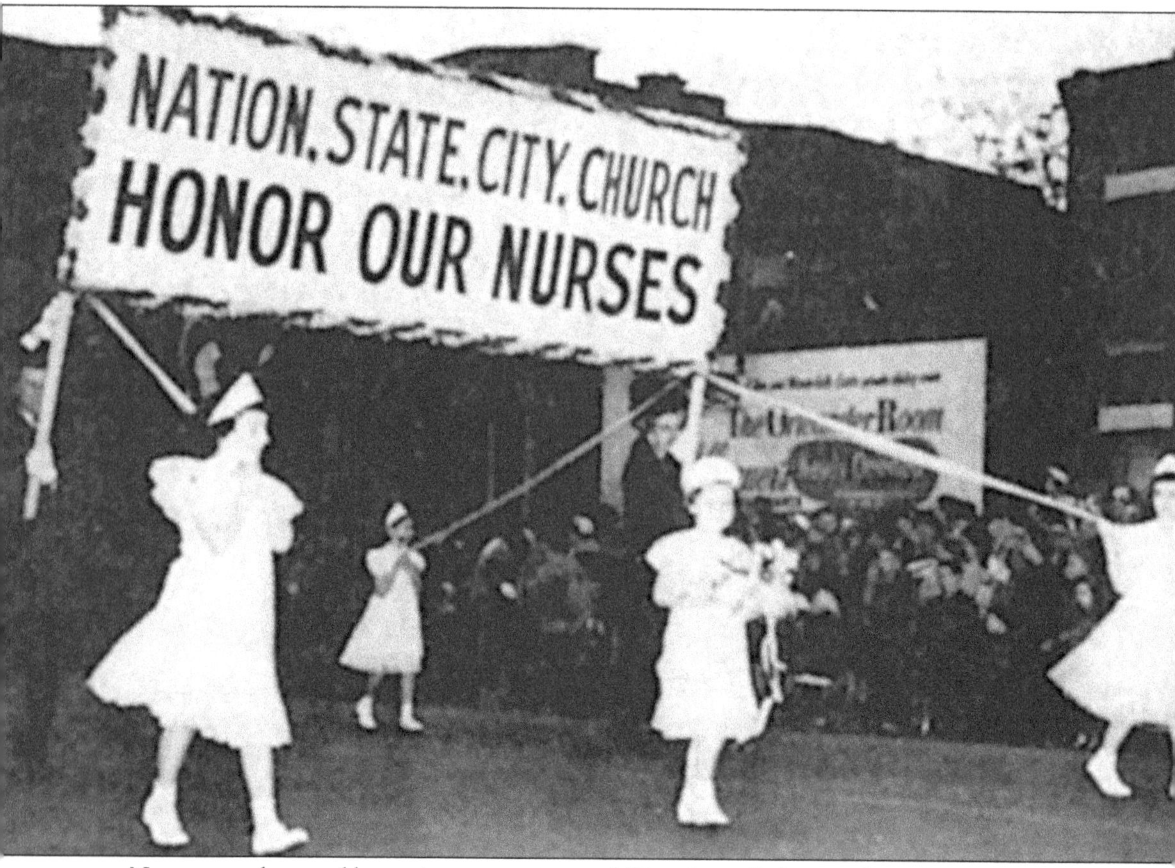

Nurses were honored by nation, state, city, and Church in all the parades. Chicago was the first city in the nation to proclaim Nurses Day and Illinois the first state. Dorothy Sutherland, of the US Department of Health, Education and Welfare, sent a proposal to President Eisenhower in 1953 for a national nurses' day to celebrate the 100th anniversary of Florence Nightingale's birth, but no action was taken. In 1974, President Nixon proclaimed National Nurse Week and in 1978, New Jersey Governor Byrne declared Nurses Day for the state. (Heather Gillies, *Today's Nurse*, April 28, 2003.) Chicago was truly in the forefront of recognizing nurses with a proclaimed day and a parade. (Image: *Novena Notes*, May 6, 1955, 13.)

Two

The Road to Success Parade Planning

Father Clarence M. Brissette recognized that there was a shortage of nurses when he was asked by many family members and patients to help them find private duty nurses. He also witnessed the caring values of nurses when he visited the sick in hospitals. He saw how hard nurses worked, the patience they exhibited, and also how tired they seemed. He took the nursing shortage into his own hands and created both Nurses Day and the Chicago Nurses Day Parade. He decided a parade would be an effective means to call attention to the need for nurses as well as to honor practicing nurses.

At its zenith, the parade drew up to 100,000 spectators and included 100 participating hospitals, 39 bands playing music, and over 4,000 uniformed nurses marching. The parade always had city and state officials in attendance; the armed forces, city police, and firemen marched as well. Most parades had a theme and the floats were decorated accordingly. Father Brissette intentionally kept the parade short "in deference to the nurses who daily pile up mileage in hospital corridors." In keeping with Father Brissette's desire to "place nursing on a national pedestal" (*New World*, 1949), red roses were placed in Our Lady of Sorrows Basilica for the services following the parade. He wanted the parade and the services to give nurses their "day of glory."

The parade was unique because merchants, government, community, religious orders, media, nursing schools, and hospitals all participated in order to make it a spectacular event. All recognized the importance of highlighting the values of nurses in a visible way. Like any major community event, the parade required planning, budgets, themes, float preparation, and cooperation from all.

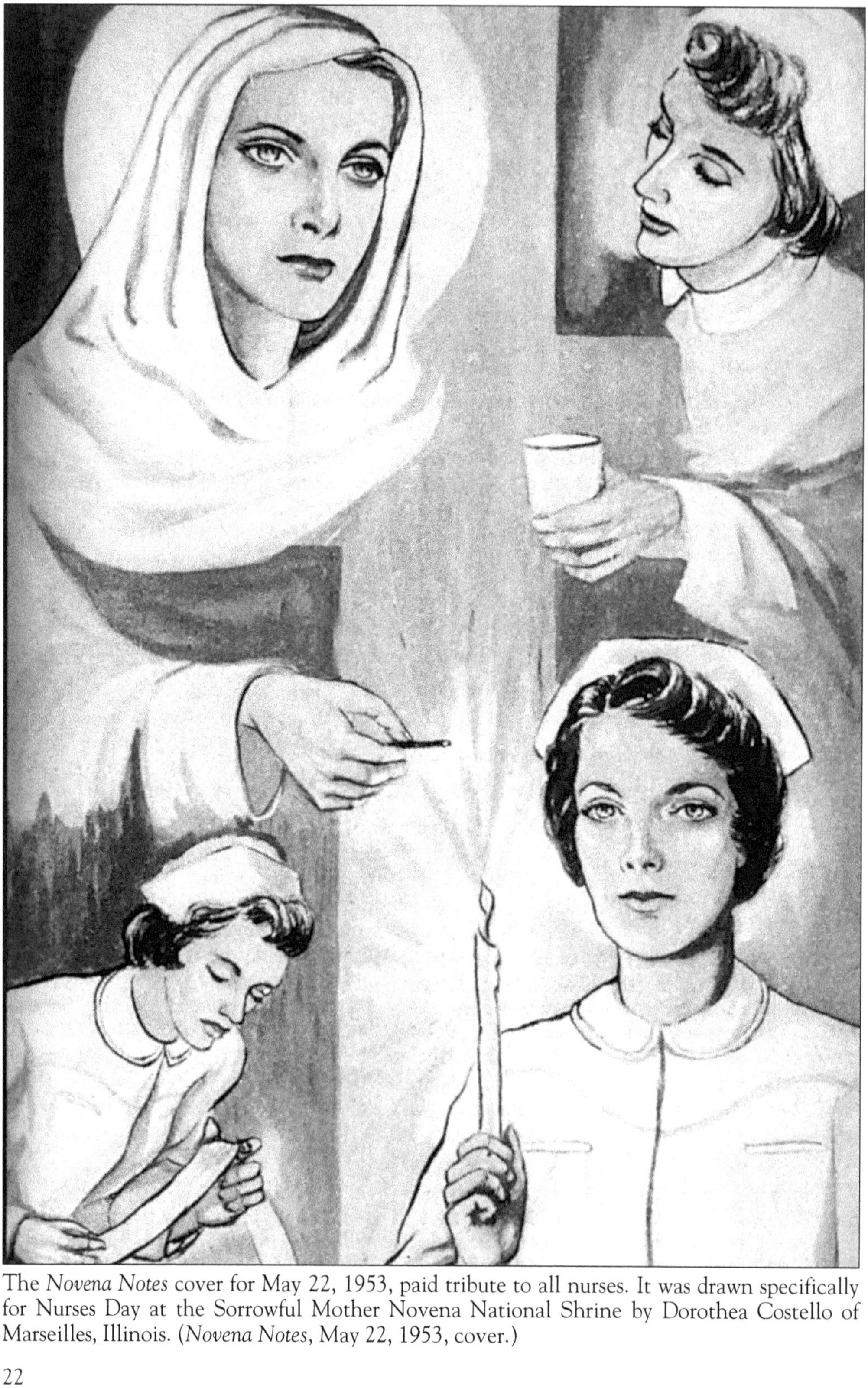

The *Novena Notes* cover for May 22, 1953, paid tribute to all nurses. It was drawn specifically for Nurses Day at the Sorrowful Mother Novena National Shrine by Dorothea Costello of Marseilles, Illinois. (*Novena Notes*, May 22, 1953, cover.)

Floats always had a theme, mostly focused on healthcare and the nurse's work. The float pictured at right was provided by Ravenswood Hospital. (*Novena Notes*, June 10, 1955, 13.)

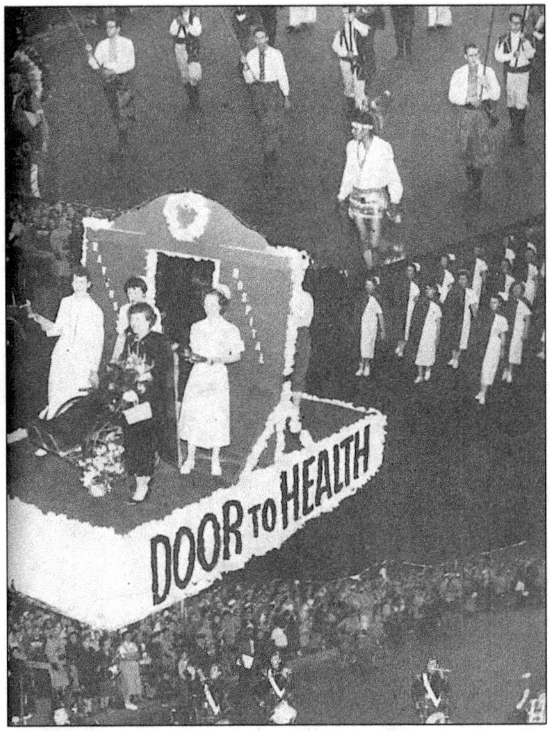

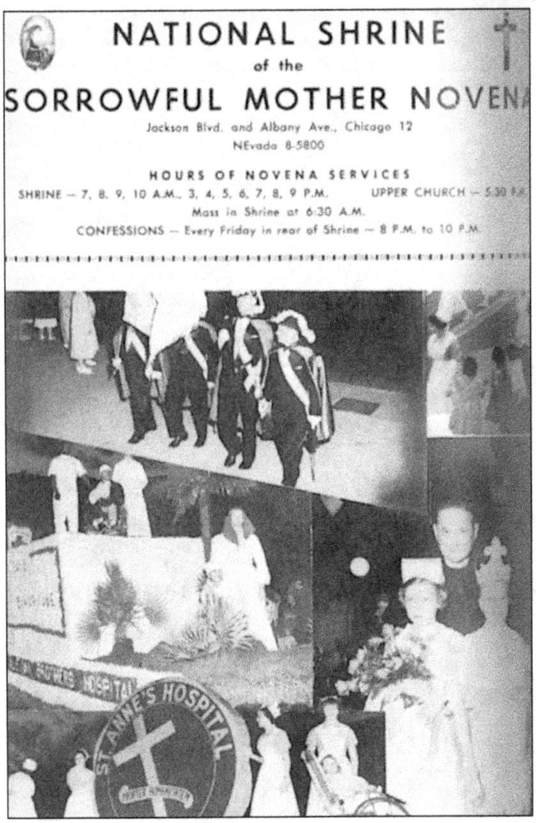
NATIONAL SHRINE
of the
SORROWFUL MOTHER NOVEN

Jackson Blvd. and Albany Ave., Chicago 12
NEvada 8-5800

HOURS OF NOVENA SERVICES
SHRINE — 7, 8, 9, 10 A.M., 3, 4, 5, 6, 7, 8, 9 P.M. UPPER CHURCH — 5:30
Mass in Shrine at 6:30 A.M.
CONFESSIONS — Every Friday in rear of Shrine — 8 P.M. to 10 P.M.

Announcements of the 1956 Nurses Parade include the name of the speaker, His Eminence Samuel Cardinal Stritch, as well as highlights from past parades. (*Novena Notes*, May 18, 1956, 2–3.)

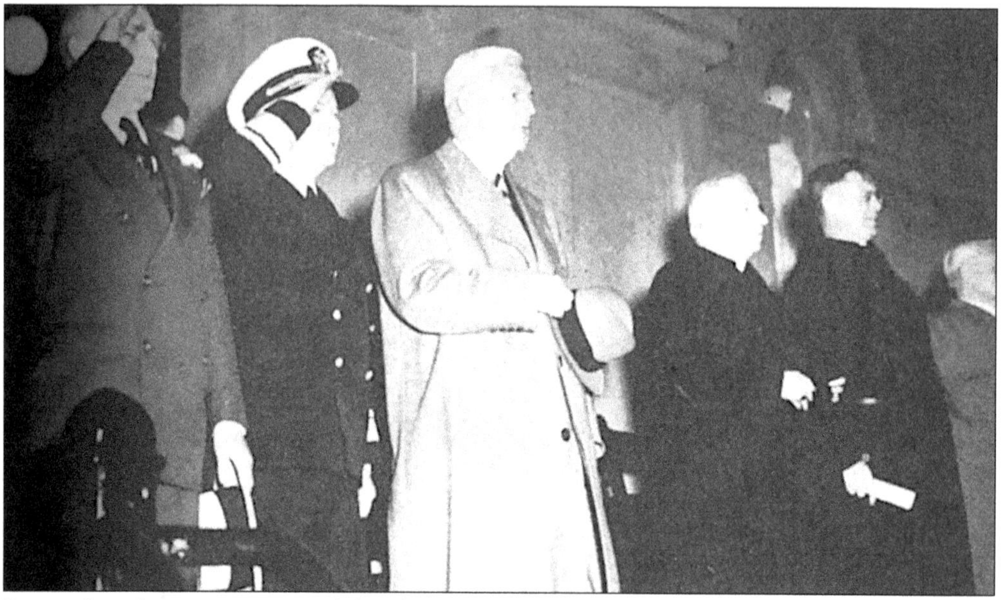

Pictured in the reviewing stand for the 1954 Nurses Day Parade, from left to right, are Dr. Herman N. Bundesen (President, Chicago Board of Health), Rear Admiral Joseph L. Kane (Grand Marshall), His Honor Martin H. Kennelly (Mayor of Chicago), His Eminence Samuel Cardinal Stritch, Very Reverend Joseph M. Srill (O.S.M., Provincial Servite American Province), and Matthew J. Corrigan (Commissioner, Chicago Fire Department). (*Novena Notes*, June 11, 1954, 3.)

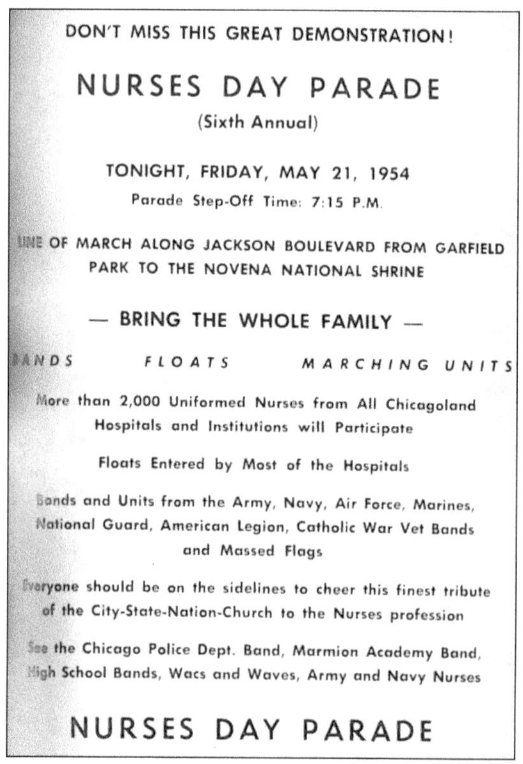
DON'T MISS THIS GREAT DEMONSTRATION!
NURSES DAY PARADE
(Sixth Annual)
TONIGHT, FRIDAY, MAY 21, 1954
Parade Step-Off Time: 7:15 P.M.
LINE OF MARCH ALONG JACKSON BOULEVARD FROM GARFIELD PARK TO THE NOVENA NATIONAL SHRINE
— BRING THE WHOLE FAMILY —
BANDS FLOATS MARCHING UNITS
More than 2,000 Uniformed Nurses from All Chicagoland Hospitals and Institutions will Participate
Floats Entered by Most of the Hospitals
Bands and Units from the Army, Navy, Air Force, Marines, National Guard, American Legion, Catholic War Vet Bands and Massed Flags
Everyone should be on the sidelines to cheer this finest tribute of the City-State-Nation-Church to the Nurses profession
See the Chicago Police Dept. Band, Marmion Academy Band, High School Bands, Wacs and Waves, Army and Navy Nurses
NURSES DAY PARADE

This is an invitation to the parade that appeared in the *Novena Notes*, May 21, 1954. The parade is often described excitedly: "Tonight is the Night. . . . Nurses Day Parade, a poetic monument to nurses, the humble, hardworking nurse, proudly, grandly marching down Jackson Boulevard. The parade, a real life fairyland, a small fragment of the nursing profession concentrated in one breathless hour of glitter and pageantry . . . casting a human, bewildering spell over an appreciative audience with eager eyes devouring, in a continual gasp of astonishment," wrote Clarence Brissette, O.S.M., Novena Director. (*Novena Notes*, May 21, 1954, 3.)

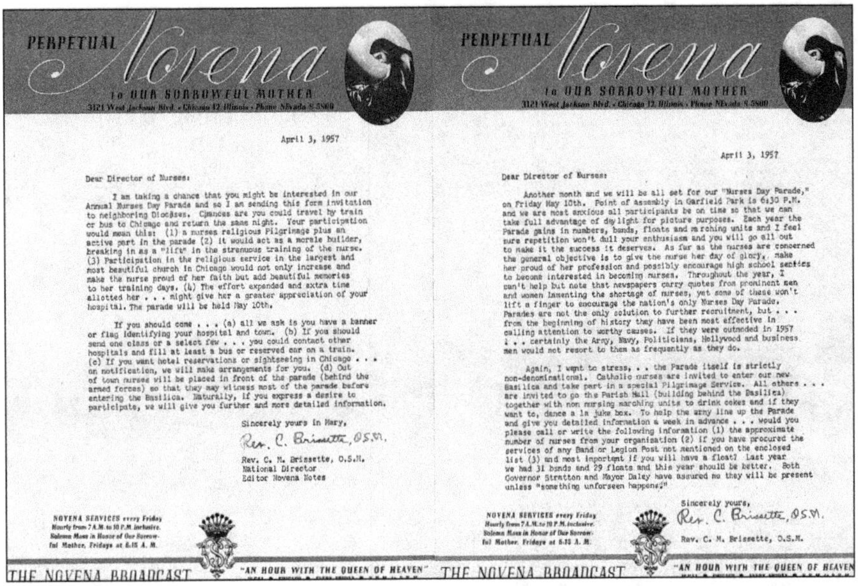

PERPETUAL Novena to OUR SORROWFUL MOTHER
3121 West Jackson Blvd. • Chicago 12 Illinois • Phone NEvada 8-5800

April 3, 1957

Dear Director of Nurses:

I am taking a chance that you might be interested in our Annual Nurses Day Parade and so I am sending this form invitation to neighboring Diocêses. Chances are you could travel by train or bus to Chicago and return the same night. Your participation would mean this: (1) a nurses religious Pilgrimage plus an active part in the parade (2) it would act as a morale builder, breaking in as a "lift" in the strenuous training of the nurse. (3) Participation in the religious service in the largest and most beautiful church in Chicago would not only increase and make the nurse proud of her faith but add beautiful memories to her training days. (4) The effort expended and extra time allotted her . . . might give her a greater appreciation of your hospital. The parade will be held May 10th.

If you should come . . . (a) all we ask is you have a banner or flag identifying your hospital and town. (b) If you should send one class or a select few . . . you could contact other hospitals and fill at least a bus or reserved car on a train. (c) If you want hotel reservations or sightseeing in Chicago . . . on notification, we will make arrangements for you. (d) Out of town nurses will be placed in front of the parade (behind the armed forces) so that they may witness most of the parade before entering the Basilica. Naturally, if you express a desire to participate, we will give you further and more detailed information.

Sincerely yours in Mary,

Rev. C. Brissette, O.S.M.

Rev. C. M. Brissette, O.S.M.
National Director
Editor Novena Notes

NOVENA SERVICES every Friday
Hourly from 7 A.M. to 10 P.M. inclusive.
Solemn Mass in Honor of Our Sorrowful Mother, Fridays at 6.15 A. M.

THE NOVENA BROADCAST "AN HOUR WITH THE QUEEN OF HEAVEN"

PERPETUAL Novena to OUR SORROWFUL MOTHER
3121 West Jackson Blvd. • Chicago 12 Illinois • Phone NEvada 8-5800

April 3, 1957

Dear Director of Nurses:

Another month and we will be all set for our "Nurses Day Parade," on Friday May 10th. Point of assembly in Garfield Park is 6:30 P.M. and we are most anxious all participants be on time so that we can take full advantage of daylight for picture purposes. Each year the Parade gains in numbers, bands, floats and marching units and I feel sure repetition won't dull your enthusiasm and you will go all out to make it the success it deserves. As far as the nurses are concerned the general objective is to give the nurse her day of glory, make her proud of her profession and possibly encourage high school seniors to become interested in becoming nurses. Throughout the year, I can't help but note that newspapers carry quotes from prominent men and women lamenting the shortage of nurses, yet some of these won't lift a finger to encourage the nation's only Nurses Day Parade. Parades are not the only solution to further recruitment, but . . . from the beginning of history they have been most effective in calling attention to worthy causes. If they were outmoded in 1957 . . . certainly the Army, Navy, Politicians, Hollywood and business men would not resort to them as frequently as they do.

Again, I want to stress, . . the Parade itself is strictly non-denominational. Catholic nurses are invited to enter our new Basilica and take part in a special Pilgrimage Service. All others . . . are invited to go the Parish Hall (building behind the Basilica) together with non nursing marching units to drink cokes and if they want to, dance a la juke box. To help the army line up the Parade and give you detailed information a week in advance . . . would you please call or write the following information (1) the approximate number of nurses from your organisation (2) if you have procured the services of any Band or Legion Post not mentioned on the enclosed list (3) and most important if you will have a float? Last year we had 31 bands and 29 floats and this year should be better. Both Governor Stratton and Mayor Daley have assured me they will be present unless "something unforseen happens."

Sincerely yours,

Rev. C. Brissette, O.S.M.

Rev. C. M. Brissette, O.S.M.

NOVENA SERVICES every Friday
Hourly from 7 A.M. to 10 P.M. inclusive.
Solemn Mass in Honor of Our Sorrowful Mother, Fridays at 6.15 A. M.

THE NOVENA BROADCAST "AN HOUR WITH THE QUEEN OF HEAVEN"

C.M. Brissette, O.S.M., national director and editor of *Novena Notes* wrote letters inviting all directors of nurses to have their nurses participate in the parade. He stressed all were welcomeand that it was strictly non-denominational. In 1958, in addition to participants in the parade, hospitals were asked to procure a band.

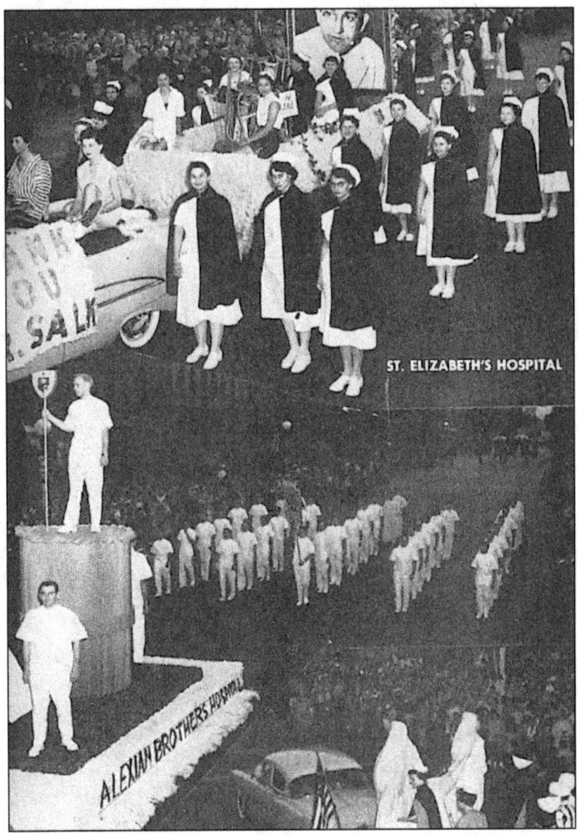

The majority of parades had a theme. At right is St. Elizabeth's hospital celebrating the work of Dr. Salk. (*Novena Notes*, June 10, 1955, 11.)

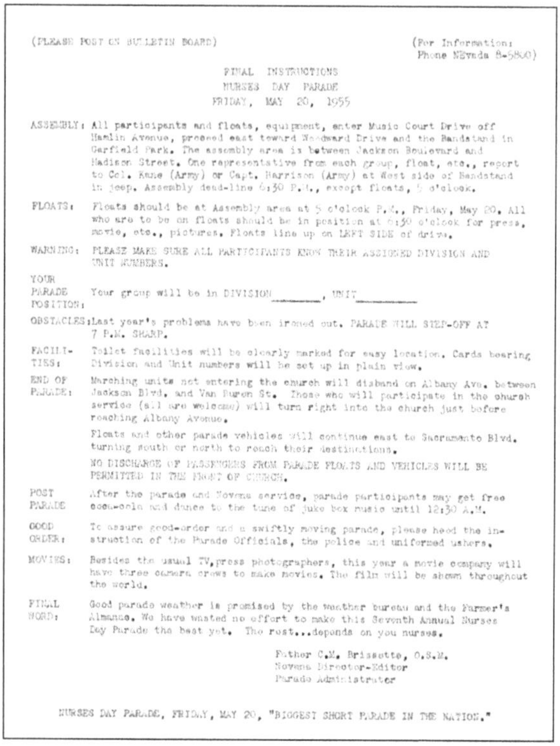

(PLEASE POST ON BULLETIN BOARD) (For Information: Phone NEvada 8-5800)

FINAL INSTRUCTIONS
NURSES DAY PARADE
FRIDAY, MAY 20, 1955

ASSEMBLY: All participants and floats, equipment, enter Music Court Drive off Hamlin Avenue, proceed east toward Woodward Drive and the Bandstand in Garfield Park. The assembly area is between Jackson Boulevard and Madison Street. One representative from each group, float, etc., report to Col. Kane (Army) or Capt. Harrison (Army) at West side of Bandstand in jeep. Assembly dead-line 6:30 P.M., except floats, 5 o'clock.

FLOATS: Floats should be at Assembly area at 5 o'clock P.M., Friday, May 20. All who are to be on floats should be in position at 6:30 o'clock for press, movie, etc., pictures. Floats line up on LEFT SIDE of drive.

WARNING: PLEASE MAKE SURE ALL PARTICIPANTS KNOW THEIR ASSIGNED DIVISION AND UNIT NUMBERS.

YOUR PARADE POSITION: Your group will be in DIVISION______, UNIT______

OBSTACLES: Last year's problems have been ironed out. PARADE WILL STEP-OFF AT 7 P.M. SHARP.

FACILITIES: Toilet facilities will be clearly marked for easy location. Cards bearing Division and Unit numbers will be set up in plain view.

END OF PARADE: Marching units not entering the church will disband on Albany Ave. between Jackson Blvd. and Van Buren St. Those who will participate in the church service (all are welcome) will turn right into the church just before reaching Albany Avenue.

Floats and other parade vehicles will continue east to Sacramento Blvd. turning south or north to reach their destinations.

NO DISCHARGE OF PASSENGERS FROM PARADE FLOATS AND VEHICLES WILL BE PERMITTED IN THE FRONT OF CHURCH.

POST PARADE: After the parade and Novena service, parade participants may get free coca-cola and dance to the tune of juke box music until 12:30 A.M.

GOOD ORDER: To assure good-order and a swiftly moving parade, please heed the instruction of the Parade Officials, the police and uniformed ushers.

MOVIES: Besides the usual TV, press photographers, this year a movie company will have three camera crews to make movies. The film will be shown throughout the world.

FINAL WORD: Good parade weather is promised by the weather bureau and the Farmer's Almanac. We have wasted no effort to make this Seventh Annual Nurses Day Parade the best yet. The rest...depends on you nurses.

Father C.M. Brissette, O.S.M.
Novena Director-Editor
Parade Administrator

NURSES DAY PARADE, FRIDAY, MAY 20, "BIGGEST SHORT PARADE IN THE NATION."

Pictured at left are the final instructions for the 1955 Nurses Day Parade. The parade took a great amount of time to plan.

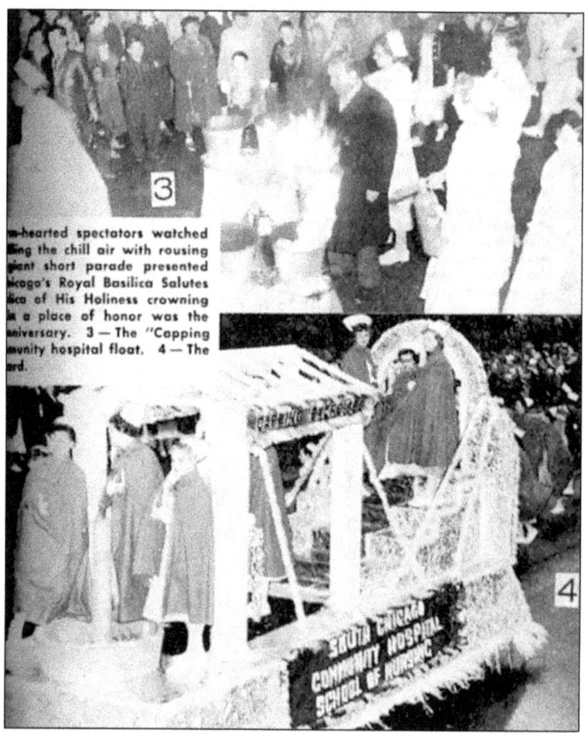
3
-hearted spectators watched
ing the chill air with rousing
ant short parade presented
icago's Royal Basilica Salutes
ica of His Holiness crowning
n a place of honor was the
niversary. 3 — The "Capping
unity hospital float. 4 — The
rd.
SOUTH CHICAGO COMMUNITY HOSPITAL SCHOOL OF NURSING
4

In 1957, the newspapers had a difficult time capturing the parade with pictures due to rain. However, WGN television showed movies of the parade the following Monday during the late-night news spot. (John Long, *Novena Notes*, May 31, 6.)

Colonial Wittacha and his aide, Captain Harrison, were in charge of lining up the nurses parade units in 1954. After the parade they were tired but happy individuals ready to do it all again in the following years. (*Novena Notes*, June 11, 1954, 2.)

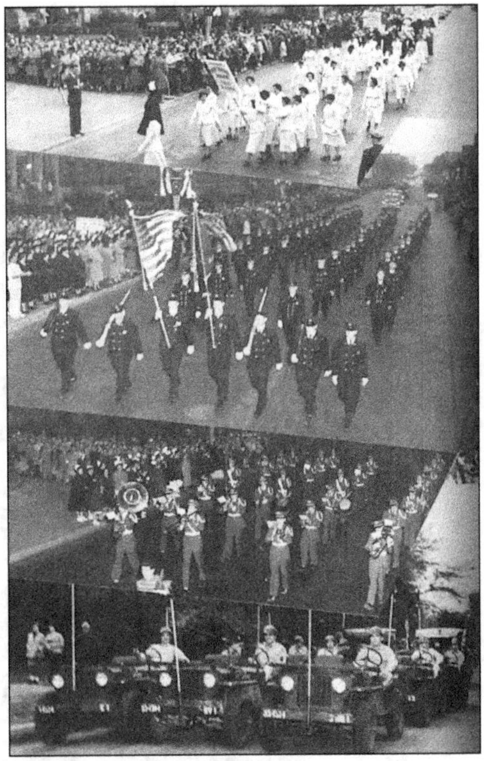

Postponed . . . to September 15th

Last year's "**Nurses' Day Parade**" was by far one of the most unique and appealing spectacles we have ever witnessed. "**Unique**" . . . by official proclamation, the first of its kind in the history of the nation! "**Appealing**" . . . the tender reaction of spectators to the magnificent sight of their "**Angels of Mercy**" on parade. At some time or other . . . the average citizen lands in some hospital . . . and then he realizes the value of the nurses and there is formed a close human bond that reveals itself when she is honored in a special way! Not long ago . . . we had a meeting of representatives from various hospitals . . . to make plans for the previously announced date for this year's "Nurses' Day." With last year's experience behind us . . . the enthusiasm displayed in making preparations, promised to exceed by five times (number of participants, floats and bands) the wonder of our first parade. There was one objection! **During the summer months, hospitals work with a skeleton force. Nurses are on vacation and many civic, military and band units are broken up for the same reason.** And again, with the opening of schools, there would be more people to witness the spectacle.

What clinched the argument was when we learned the Illinois National Guard would be in training. (Last year the Army headed the parade with the Black Horse Troop, a band, three army units and eight ambulances.) Considering everything . . . we decided to postpone "**Nurses' Day" until September 15th!** **St. Camillus,** first to use the Red Cross and universal patron of hospitals and nurses, will still be honored. (His Feast Day is in July . . . the reason why we originally picked this month to honor nurses.) So . . . **Chicagoans, visitors, and out-of-town hospitals (who might want to participate) make your plans for the early evening of September 15th.** If anyone . . . wants to make a week-end pilgrimage of the occasion, contact **Gibbs Tours, 220 S. State Street, Chicago 4, Illinois** and make arrangements now!

Due to school vacations and the shortage of nurses, the 1950 parade was postponed to the fall. (*Novena Notes*, July 7, 1950, back cover.)

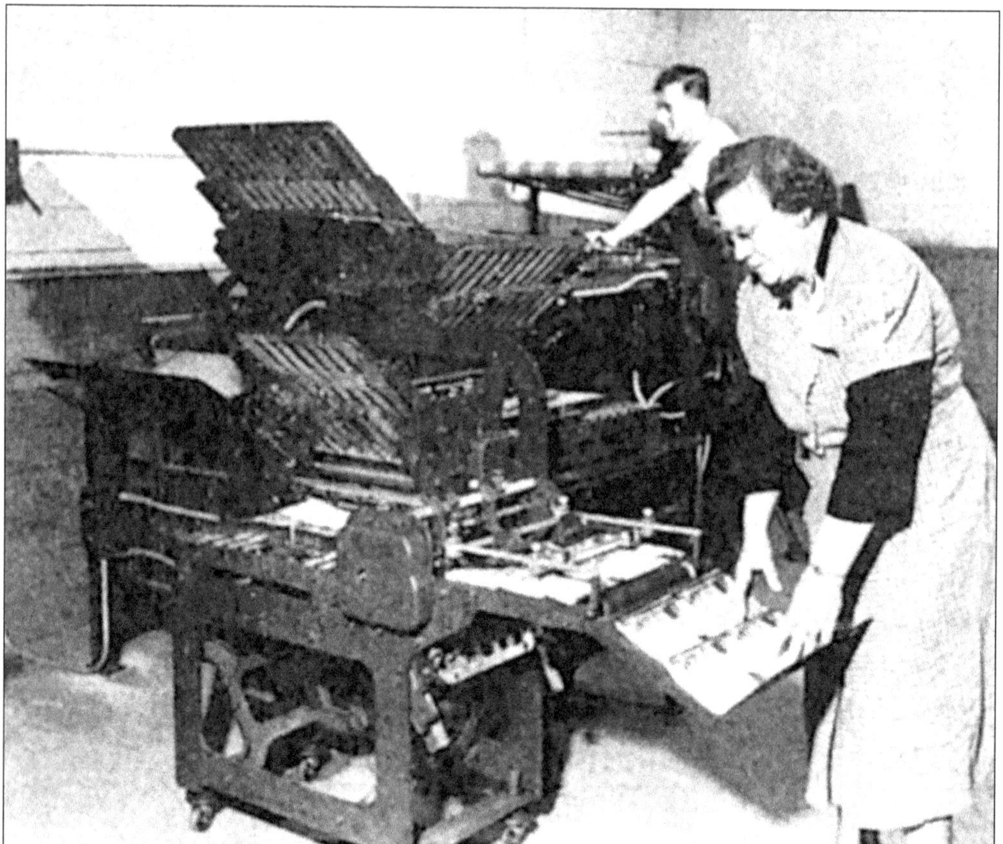

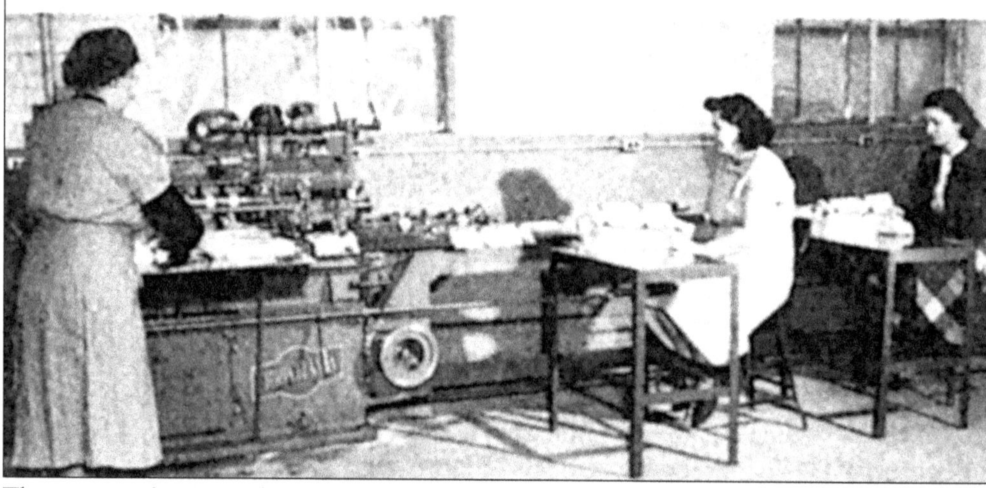

The process of printing the *Novena Notes*, which used the most "up-to-date" equipment in the 1940s, is seen above and opposite here. The majority of images from this book and the history of the parade come from the *Novena Notes*, archived at Our Lady of Sorrows Basilica.

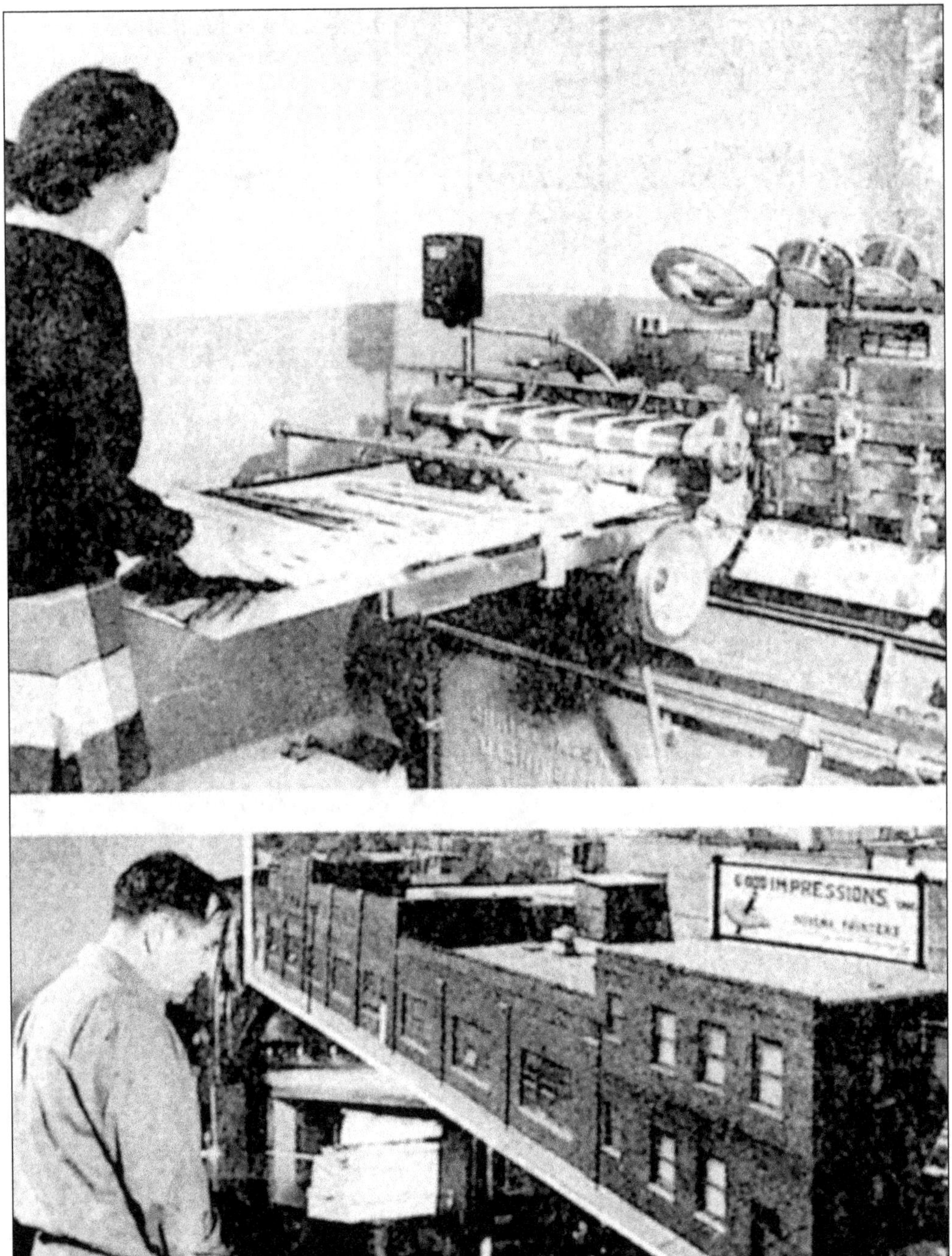

Father Conrad Borntrager graciously granted permission to reproduce these images along with other images in the book. (*Novena Notes*, August 12, 1949, 8–9.)

Morris B. Sachs Inc.

SOUTH—6638 SOUTH HALSTED STREET • NORTH—3400 DIVERSEY AVENUE

CHICAGO

EXECUTIVE OFFICE
6638 S. HALSTED ST.
CHICAGO 21, ILLINOIS

April 5, 1957

Reverend Clarence Brissette
Our Lady of Sorrows Church
3121 West Jackson Blvd.
Chicago, Illinois

Dear Father Brissette:

Enclosed is my check for $500.00, which I hope will help in your endeavor.

God bless you, and with my kindest personal regards, I am

Sincerely,

Morris B. Sachs

MBS:jk
Enc.

Chicago merchants assisted in financing the Nurses Day Parades.

PERPETUAL Novena
to OUR SORROWFUL MOTHER
3121 West Jackson Blvd. - Chicago 12, Illinois - Phone NEvada 8-5800

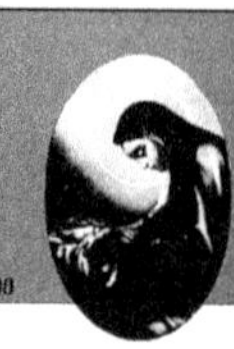

Dear Director of Nurses:

Every so often . . . men and women representing public relations, paid to publicize hospitals get their names in print and most often their song and dance accents the great shortage of nurses. While the public weeps . . . I check on the record and find the same do little toward making Nurses Day the success it should be. Parades are not the only answer to recruiting, but . . . thousands of years B.C. parades were used as morale builders and also to call attention to definite needs.

This is our 10th Anniversary and I hope in scope and beauty the Parade on May 9th lives up the part. Regardless of religious affiliation . . . the primary purpose of the parade is to give the Nurse a lift, make her proud of her profession and to encourage recruitment. If for some reason or other, your hospital will not take part in an official way . . . would you please place the accompanying poster in a conspicuous place and at least make the information available to your Nurses. Again I assure you the parade is non-denominational and that I am a simple priest who recognized a need for more nurses and tried to do something about it. We welcome anyone identified with the nursing profession provided they have uniforms such as Nurses Aides etc.

This year I am a little short on funds and have three American Legion organizations with the slogan: "have band, will march." If any one hospital would like to help and contribute bus transportation for one band notify me immediately so that I can enjoy the prospect of spending the week following the parade out of jail. Please call the Novena Office before Saturday May 3rd and let me know (1) approximate number of nurses that will march (2) if you will have a float or (3) band and I will send you the order of the parade the early part of next week.

Sincerely yours,

Rev. C. Brissette, O.S.M.

NOVENA SERVICES every Friday
Hourly from 7 A.M. to 10 P.M. inclusive.
Solemn Mass in Honor of Our Sorrowful Mother, Fridays at 6:15 A. M.

THE NOVENA BROADCAST "AN HOUR WITH THE QUEEN OF HEAVEN"
WCFL • CHICAGO • EVERY FRIDAY • 8 P. M. to 9 P. M.

This is a letter inviting participation and support for the 10th Anniversary of the Chicago Nurses Day Parade, which was short of funds.

The 1956 Nurses Day Parade balance sheet showed a deficit of $978.

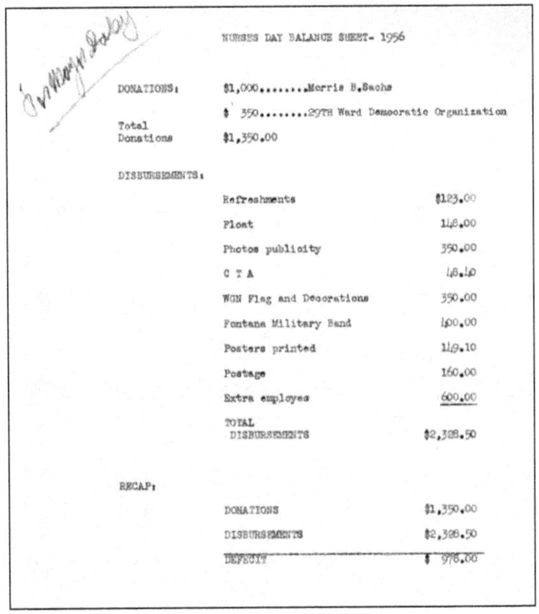

NURSES DAY BALANCE SHEET- 1956

DONATIONS: $1,000........Morris B.Sachs

$ 350........29TH Ward Democratic Organization

Total Donations $1,350.00

DISBURSEMENTS:

Refreshments	$123.00
Float	148.00
Photos publicity	350.00
C T A	48.40
WGN Flag and Decorations	350.00
Fontana Military Band	400.00
Posters printed	149.10
Postage	160.00
Extra employes	600.00
TOTAL DISBURSEMENTS	$2,328.50

RECAP:

DONATIONS	$1,350.00
DISBURSEMENTS	$2,328.50
DEFECIT	$ 978.00

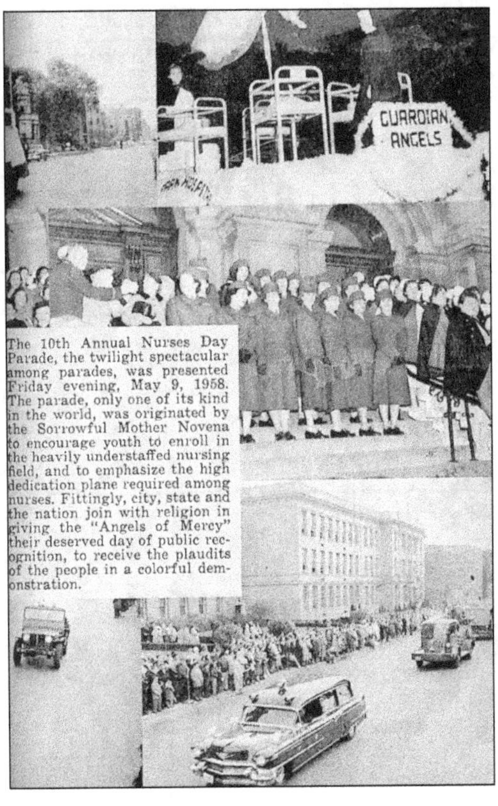
GUARDIAN ANGELS
The 10th Annual Nurses Day Parade, the twilight spectacular among parades, was presented Friday evening, May 9, 1958. The parade, only one of its kind in the world, was originated by the Sorrowful Mother Novena to encourage youth to enroll in the heavily understaffed nursing field, and to emphasize the high dedication plane required among nurses. Fittingly, city, state and the nation join with religion in giving the "Angels of Mercy" their deserved day of public recognition, to receive the plaudits of the people in a colorful demonstration.

In 1958, the theme for the parade was "Student Nurses." Father Brissette was out of town until Easter of that year and needed help in planning the parade. For the first time he developed a parade planning committee. The chairperson was Hedwig M. Weiler, R.N., from Norwegian American Hospital. (*Novena Notes*, May 30, 1958, 9.)

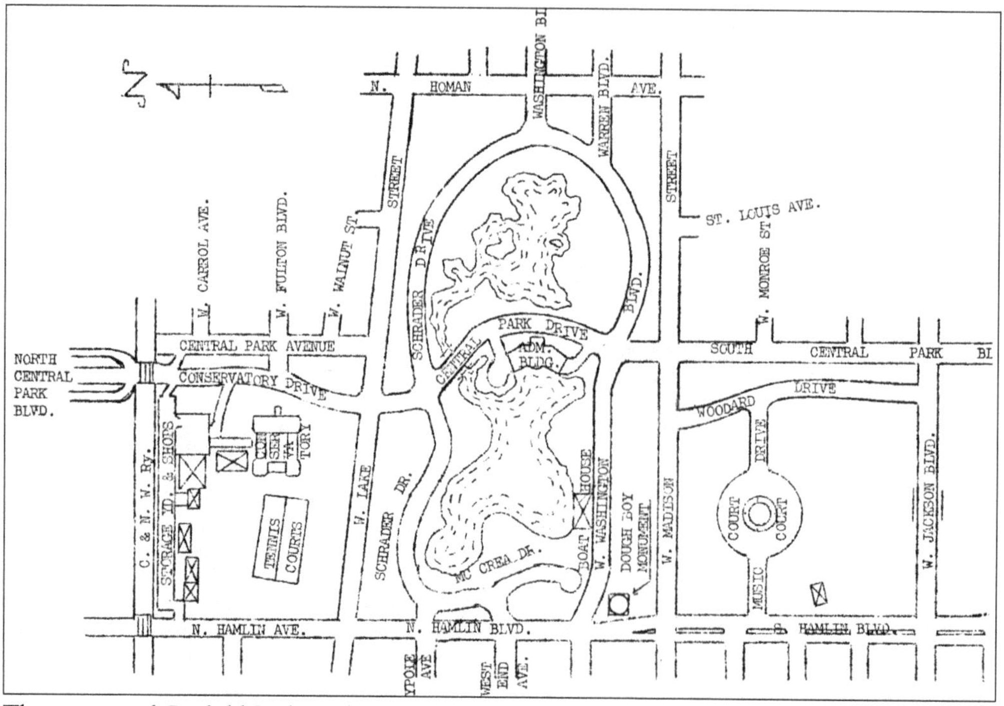

The section of Garfield Park to the right was the staging area for the parade, which proceeded along Jackson Boulevard to Albany Avenue. The parade was described as the "world's largest, shortest parade." Father Brissette thought nurses put on a lot of miles in the hospital halls and did not want them to tire in the parade. The parade was six blocks in length and lasted one hour.

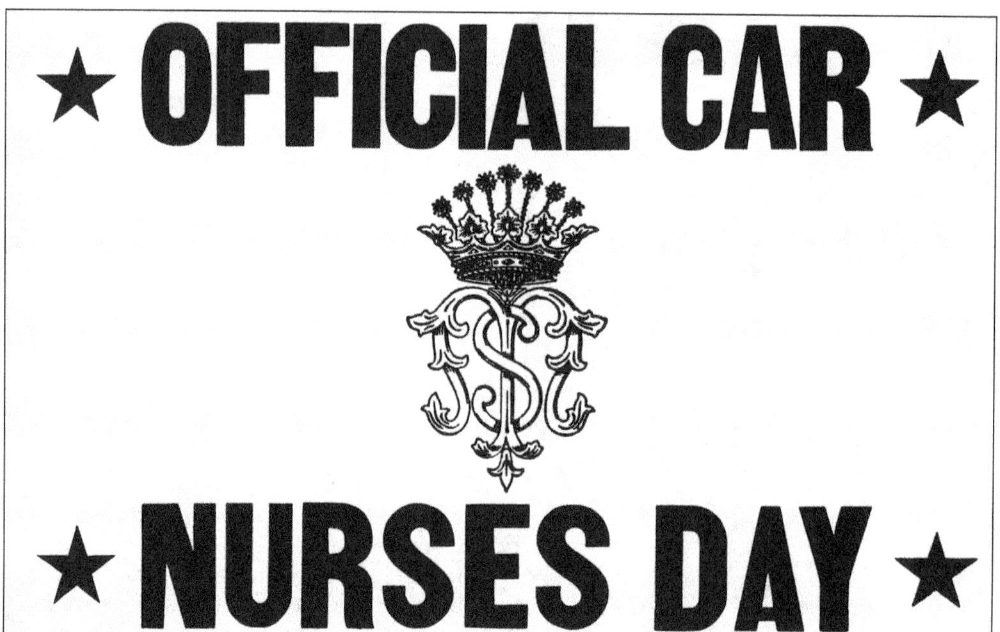

A Nurses Day official car sign is seen here. It serves as another example of the City of Chicago being a true partner and supporter of the Nurses Day Parade.

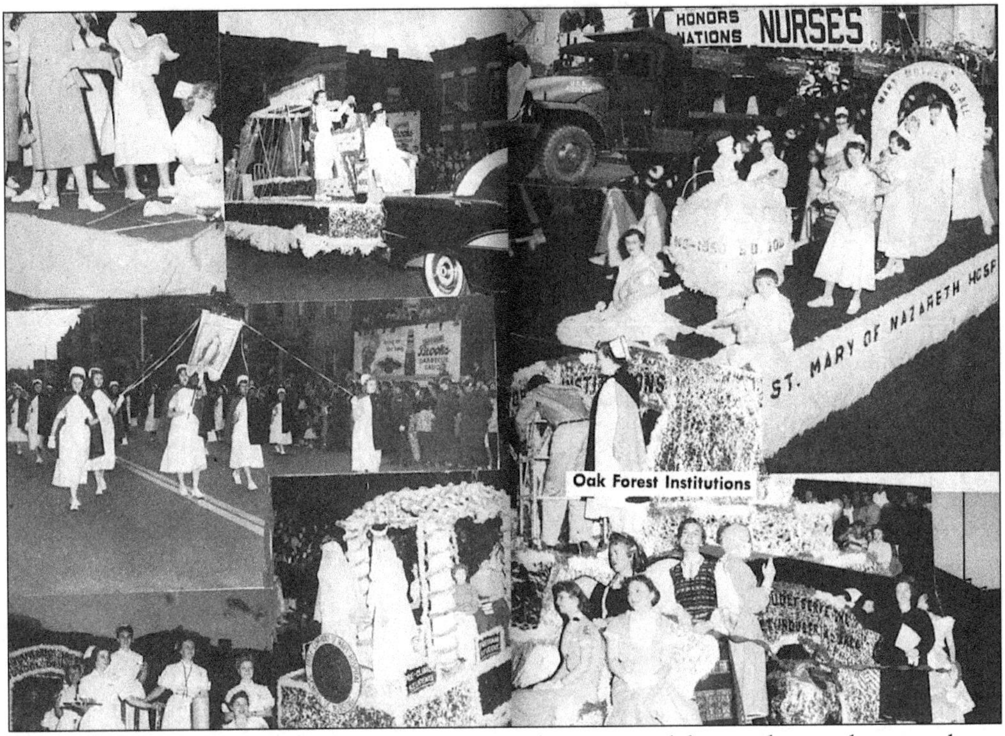

President Eisenhower's tight schedule did not permit him to attend the parade, stated a press release. The president expressed his regret and voiced "his deep admiration for the nursing profession," which he "holds it in great respect and esteem." (*Novena Notes*, June 8, 1956, 12–13.)

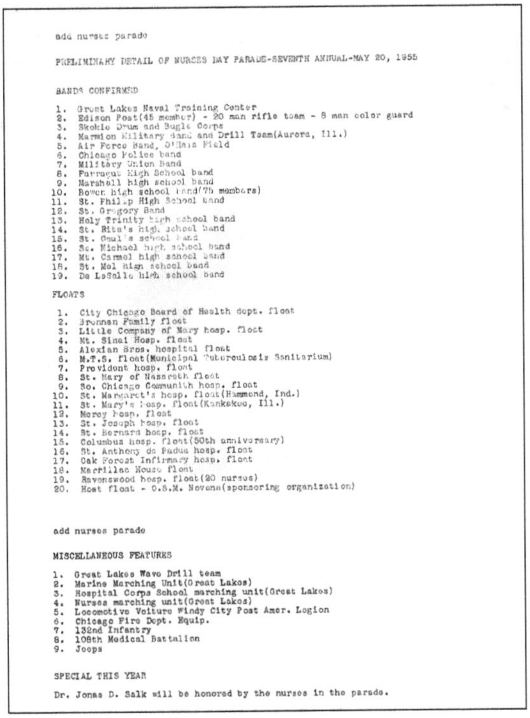

add nurses parade

PRELIMINARY DETAIL OF NURSES DAY PARADE-SEVENTH ANNUAL-MAY 20, 1955

BANDS CONFIRMED

1. Great Lakes Naval Training Center
2. Edison Post(45 member) - 20 man rifle team - 8 man color guard
3. Skokie Drum and Bugle Corps
4. Marmion Military Band and Drill Team(Aurora, Ill.)
5. Air Force Band, O'Hare Field
6. Chicago Police band
7. Military Union Band
8. Farragut High School band
9. Marshall high school band
10. Bowen high school band(75 members)
11. St. Philip High School band
12. St. Gregory Band
13. Holy Trinity high school band
14. St. Rita's high school band
15. St. Gaul's school band
16. St. Michael high school band
17. Mt. Carmel high school band
18. St. Mel high school band
19. De LaSalle high school band

FLOATS

1. City Chicago Board of Health dept. float
2. Brennan Family float
3. Little Company of Mary hosp. float
4. Mt. Sinai Hosp. float
5. Alexian Bros. hospital float
6. M.T.S. float(Municipal Tuberculosis Sanitarium)
7. Provident hosp. float
8. St. Mary of Nazareth float
9. So. Chicago Communith hosp. float
10. St. Margaret's hosp. float(Hammond, Ind.)
11. St. Mary's hosp. float(Kankakee, Ill.)
12. Mercy hosp. float
13. St. Joseph hosp. float
14. St. Bernard hosp. float
15. Columbus hosp. float(50th anniversary)
16. St. Anthony de Padua hosp. float
17. Oak Forest Infirmary hosp. float
18. Marillac House float
19. Ravenswood hosp. float(20 nurses)
20. Host float - O.S.M. Novena(sponsoring organization)

add nurses parade

MISCELLANEOUS FEATURES

1. Great Lakes Wave Drill team
2. Marine Marching Unit(Great Lakes)
3. Hospital Corps School marching unit(Great Lakes)
4. Nurses marching unit(Great Lakes)
5. Locomotive Voiture Windy City Post Amer. Legion
6. Chicago Fire Dept. Equip.
7. 132nd Infantry
8. 108th Medical Battalion
9. Joops

SPECIAL THIS YEAR

Dr. Jonas D. Salk will be honored by the nurses in the parade.

This document contains some of the details for the Seventh Annual Chicago Nurses Day Parade.

From the Desk of

TOM SEERY

PIX NOTE FOR MAY 15 A M

Mayor Daley will receive Father C.M.Brissette, O.S.M. director of the Sorrowful Mother Novena sponsors of the 8TH Annual Nurses Day parade (May 18), in the City Hall Tuesday (May 15) morning at 10:15 o'clock to review final plans for the public tribute in honor of nurses, only one of its kind in the nation. At the same time Mayor Daley will accept the invitation and honor to serve as "Grand Marshal" of the parade.

xxx

Mayor Richard J. Daley accepted the invitation to be the parade's "Grand Marshal" in 1956.

RICHARD J. DALEY
MAYOR

CITY OF CHICAGO
OFFICE OF THE MAYOR

April 12, 1956

Dear Friend:

May 18 has been proclaimed "Nurses Day in Chicago." As in years past, the occasion will be marked by a Nurses' Parade under the sponsorship of the Novena to Our Sorrowful Mother.

~~I have been informed that~~ this annual parade serves as an effective means of drawing attention to the vital need for trained nurses and as an incentive for the enlistment of recruits for this humanitarian service, the dedicated profession of nursing.

It has been also brought to my attention that this year's parade coincides with the closing of the national convention of the American Association of Nurses, which this year will be held in Chicago.

It would seem most fitting that all nursing units in the Chicago area join in making this parade of impressive significance for the nation.

Sincerely,

Richard J. Daley

MAYOR

Mayor Daley supported the parade and supported nurses. He believed the parade drew attention to the need for more nurses.

Mayor Daley, Grand Marshal of the Annual Nurses Day Parade, is pictured here in 1957 talking over the line-up with Father Brissette, director of the Sorrowful Mother Novena, while holding the poster announcing the parade. The parade started at 7 p.m. on Friday night, May 10th at Garfield Park and moved eastward to Albany Avenue. (*Novena Notes*, May 3, 1957, 16.)

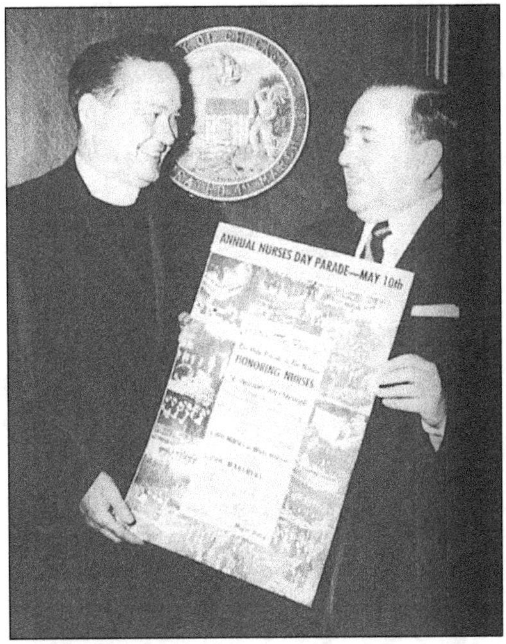

CHICAGO PARK DISTRICT

TRAFFIC SECTION · ENGINEERING DIVISION

6TH ANNUAL NURSES' DAY PARADE

SPONSORED BY — The Sorrowful Mother Novena. For further information contact The Reverend Clarence M. Brissette, O.S.M., telephone Nevada 8-5800.

DATE AND TIME — Friday, May 20, 1955.

Assembly will start at 6:30 P.M.

Parade will start at 7:00 P.M. promptly.

ATTENDANCE — It is anticipated that approximately 4,000 marchers including Nurses, Firemen, Army, Navy, Marine and Illinois National Guard Units and Bands, American Legion Posts, Veterans of Foreign Wars, Amvets, Catholic War Veterans and High School Bands will participate in the parade, also approximately 25 floats.

ASSEMBLY — Colonel Francis P. Kane, Illinois National Guard, in charge assisted by Captain James W. Harrison.

Assembly will be on Woodward and Music Court Drives in Garfield Park. Entrance to area for all participants and floats will be at Music Court Drive and Hamlin Boulevard.

LINE OF MARCH — The line of march will be from Woodward Drive, east on Jackson Boulevard to Albany Avenue.

DISBANDING — Those marchers participating in the parade attending the services at Our Lady of Sorrows Church will enter the church direct from the parade but in such a manner as to not hold up the parade.

Those marching units not attending the services will disband on Albany Avenue between Jackson Boulevard and Van Buren Street.

Floats and other vehicles in the parade leaving the area immediately will continue east to Sacramento Boulevard and on to their destinations either north or south.

NO FLOATS WILL BE PERMITTED TO DISCHARGE THEIR PASSENGERS IMMEDIATELY IN FRONT OF THE CHURCH BUT WILL DO SO ALONG THE CURBS EAST OF ALBANY AVENUE OR ON VAN BUREN STREET.

REROUTING OF TRAFFIC — At 7:00 A.M. Woodward Drive will be closed to traffic at Madison Street and Jackson Boulevard and Music Court Drive at Hamlin Boulevard.

At 6:45 P.M., or as soon as necessary, eastbound Jackson Boulevard traffic will be detoured north and south on Hamlin Boulevard.

At 6:45 P.M., or as soon as necessary, westbound Jackson Boulevard traffic will be detoured north and south at Sacramento Boulevard.

(Continued)

6th Annual Nurses' Day Parade (Continued)

2.

SPECIAL BARRICADES AND SIGNS — The TRAFFIC SECTION, ENGINEERING DIVISION will close Woodward Drive at Madison Street and at Jackson Boulevard and Music Court Drive at Hamlin Avenue not later than 7:00 A.M., Friday, May 20, 1955. Drives to remain closed until parade leaves the assembly area.

"No Parking between 4:00 P.M. and 9:00 P.M." signs will be erected along both curbs of Jackson Boulevard between Central Park Boulevard and Sacramento Boulevard not later than 7:00 A.M., Friday, May 20, 1955.

MAINTENANCE OF ORDER AND PROTECTION — The CHICAGO PARK DISTRICT POLICE DIVISION will have sufficient police along the line of march to direct and control traffic and pedestrian movements.

Arrangements have been made with the Police of the City of Chicago to allow no private vehicular traffic to proceed south of Fifth Avenue or north of Van Buren Street on Kedzie Avenue, southwest of Adams Street on Fifth Avenue or south of Adams Street or north of Van Buren Street on Homan Avenue and northeast on Fifth Avenue from Central Park Avenue. Public transportation vehicles will be permitted through these points at all times, however, and will break through the parade at intervals.

REMARKS — The sponsor of this event should call Harrison 7-1190 immediately, if any emergency arises necessitating a revision of the schedule herein listed.

Traffic Section: Richard G. Fencl, Traffic Engineer

Police Division: George A. Otlewis, Chief of Police

Approved: George T. Donoghue, General Superintendent

S-7
RFB.fcr
Copies to General Mailing List
May 12, 1955

For further traffic details contact the Traffic Engineer.

Extensive planning took place for every parade since it was necessary to utilize a lot of Chicago resources, including the police and the Chicago Park District.

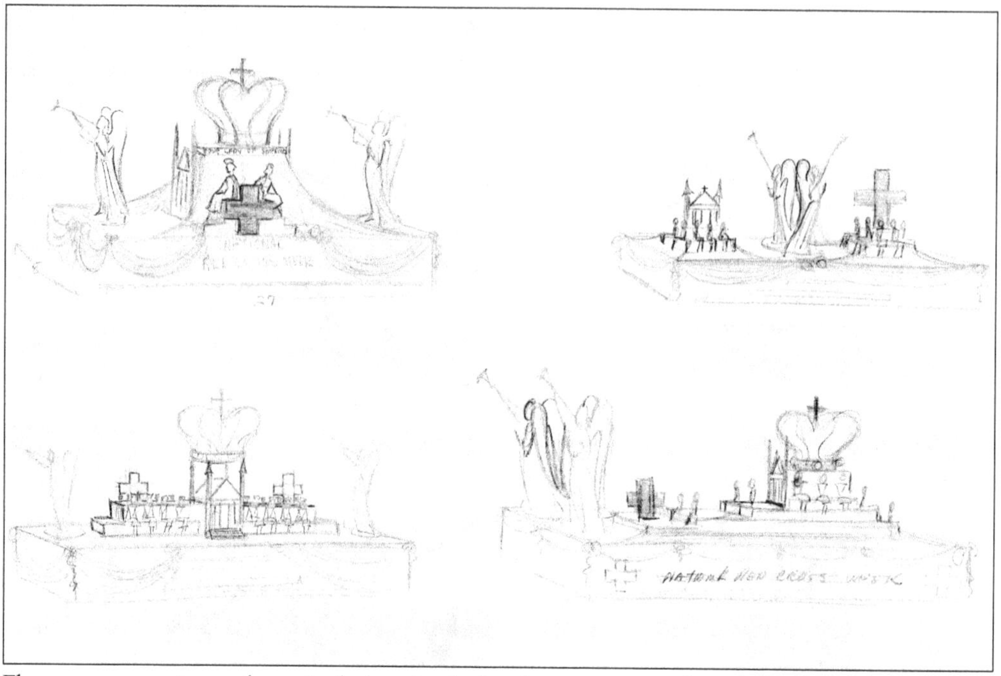

Floats were creative and required planning before becoming a reality in the parade.

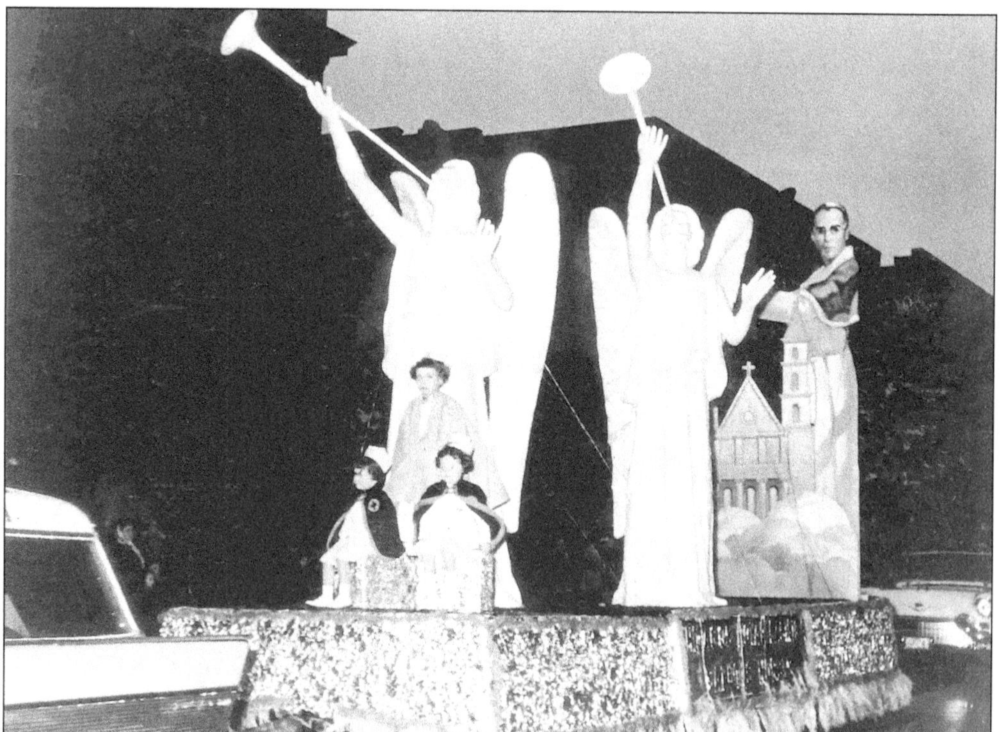

A float highlighting the Red Cross symbol came alive during the parade after it had been sketched and thoughtfully designed. This Novena float leads the 1957 parade, highlighting National Red Cross Week.

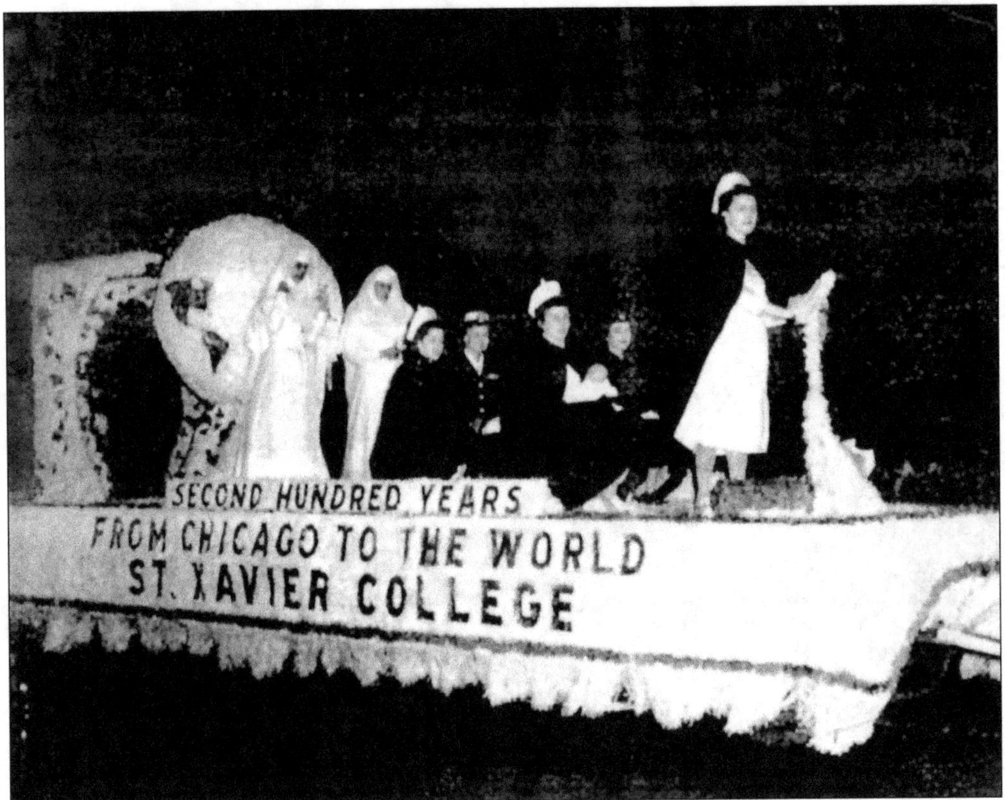

St. Xavier College participated in the Ninth Annual Nurses Day Parade. The school had been established in 1889 and was the oldest in Illinois. In 1957, St. Xavier College was 68 years old. The float theme was "around the world in 68 years."

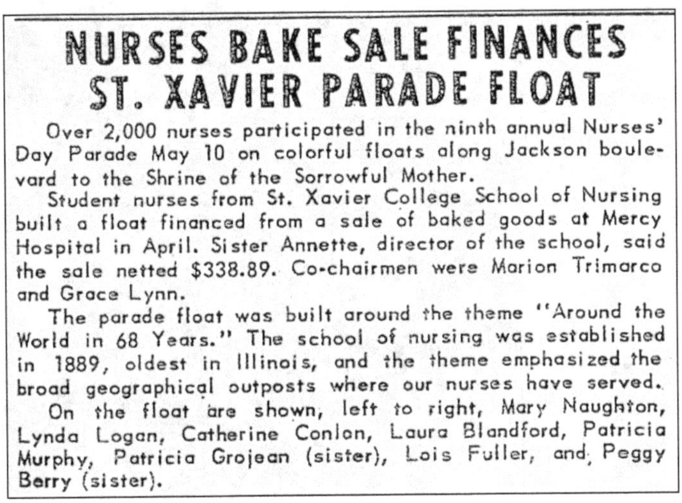

NURSES BAKE SALE FINANCES ST. XAVIER PARADE FLOAT

Over 2,000 nurses participated in the ninth annual Nurses' Day Parade May 10 on colorful floats along Jackson boulevard to the Shrine of the Sorrowful Mother.

Student nurses from St. Xavier College School of Nursing built a float financed from a sale of baked goods at Mercy Hospital in April. Sister Annette, director of the school, said the sale netted $338.89. Co-chairmen were Marion Trimarco and Grace Lynn.

The parade float was built around the theme "Around the World in 68 Years." The school of nursing was established in 1889, oldest in Illinois, and the theme emphasized the broad geographical outposts where our nurses have served.

On the float are shown, left to right, Mary Naughton, Lynda Logan, Catherine Conlon, Laura Blandford, Patricia Murphy, Patricia Grojean (sister), Lois Fuller, and Peggy Berry (sister).

This is a story about St. Xavier participants in the ninth annual parade. Their float was funded by a bake sale that was held at Mercy Hospital. The donations from the bake sale totaled $338.89.

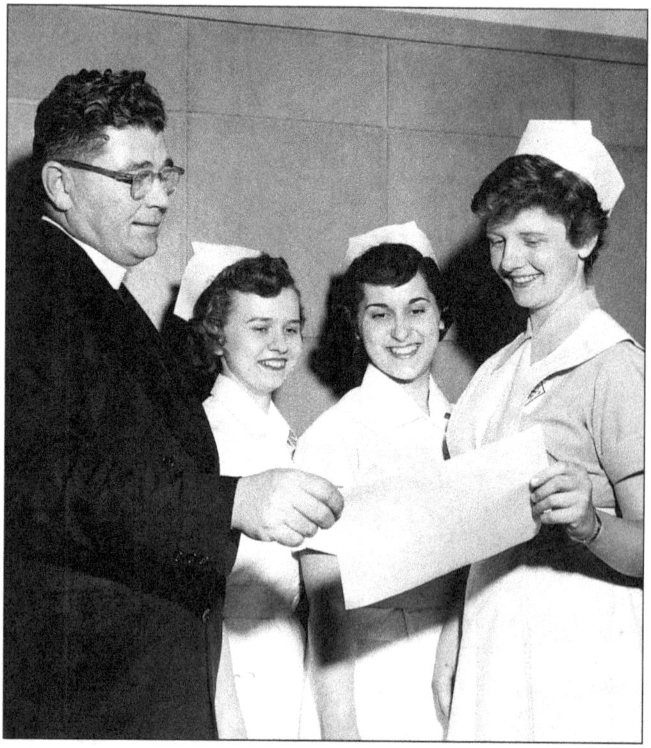

Here, nurses prepare for the 1956 parade. This photo appeared in the *Chicago Daily News* on May 16, 1956, featuring Father John M. Wondrasek, O.S.M., assistant director of the Sorrowful Mother Novena. The designers of the winning float are from St. Anne's Hospital. Pictured here are Susan Radek of Lombard (right), Marion Tyson of Newcastle (left), and Susan Barbata of Chicago (center).

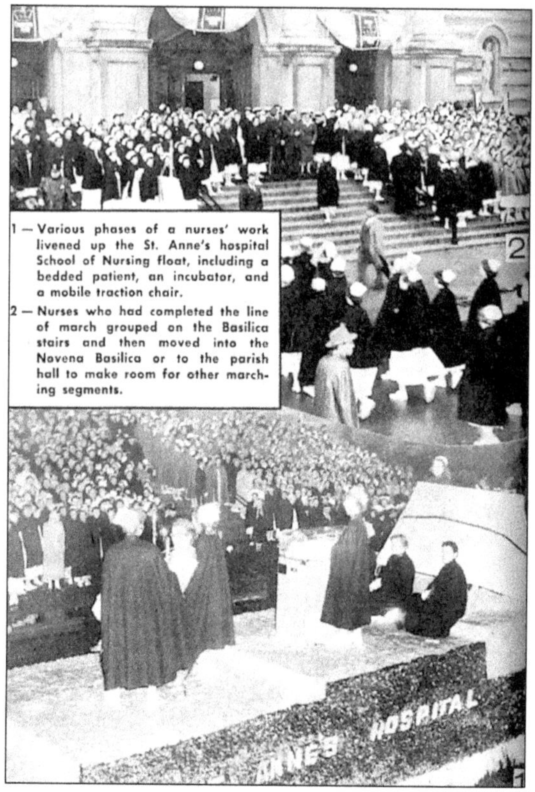

After the parade ended in 1957, nurses started planning for the following year. They did not know at the time that it would be the last one. (John Long, *Novena Notes*, May 31, 1957, 6.)

Float preparation and planning was appreciated by spectators, who demonstrated by cheering. (*Novena Notes*, June 10, 1955, 14.)

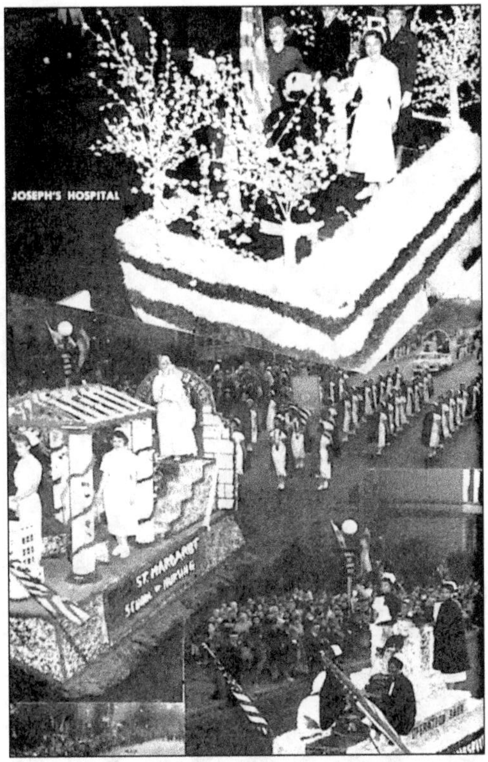

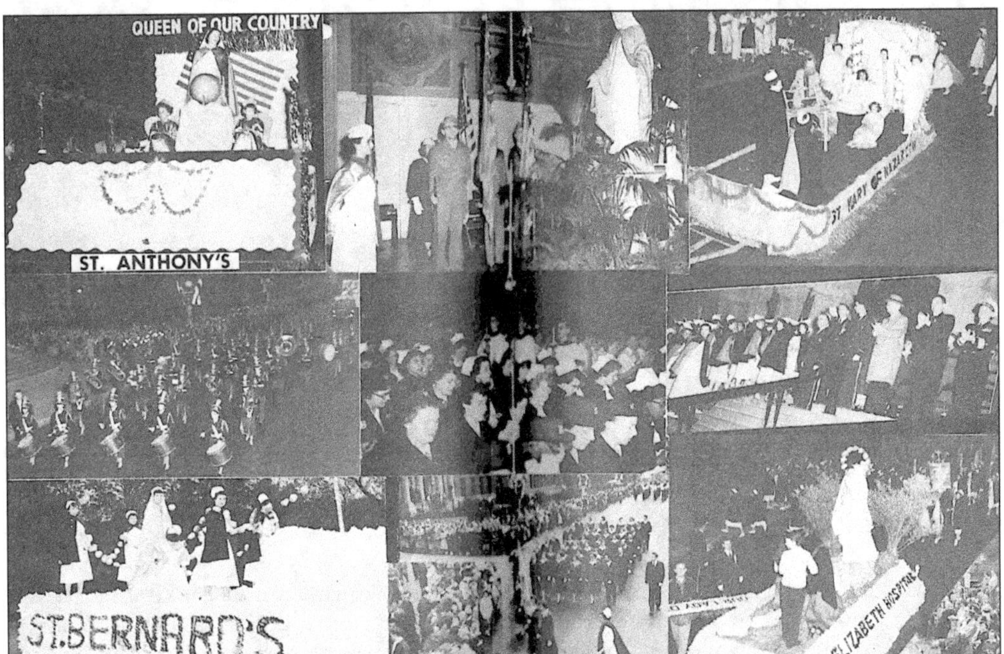

Chicago Park District officials and the media declared the Nurses Day Parade on par with any parade held on Michigan Avenue. (*Novena Notes*, June 11, 1954, 7–8.)

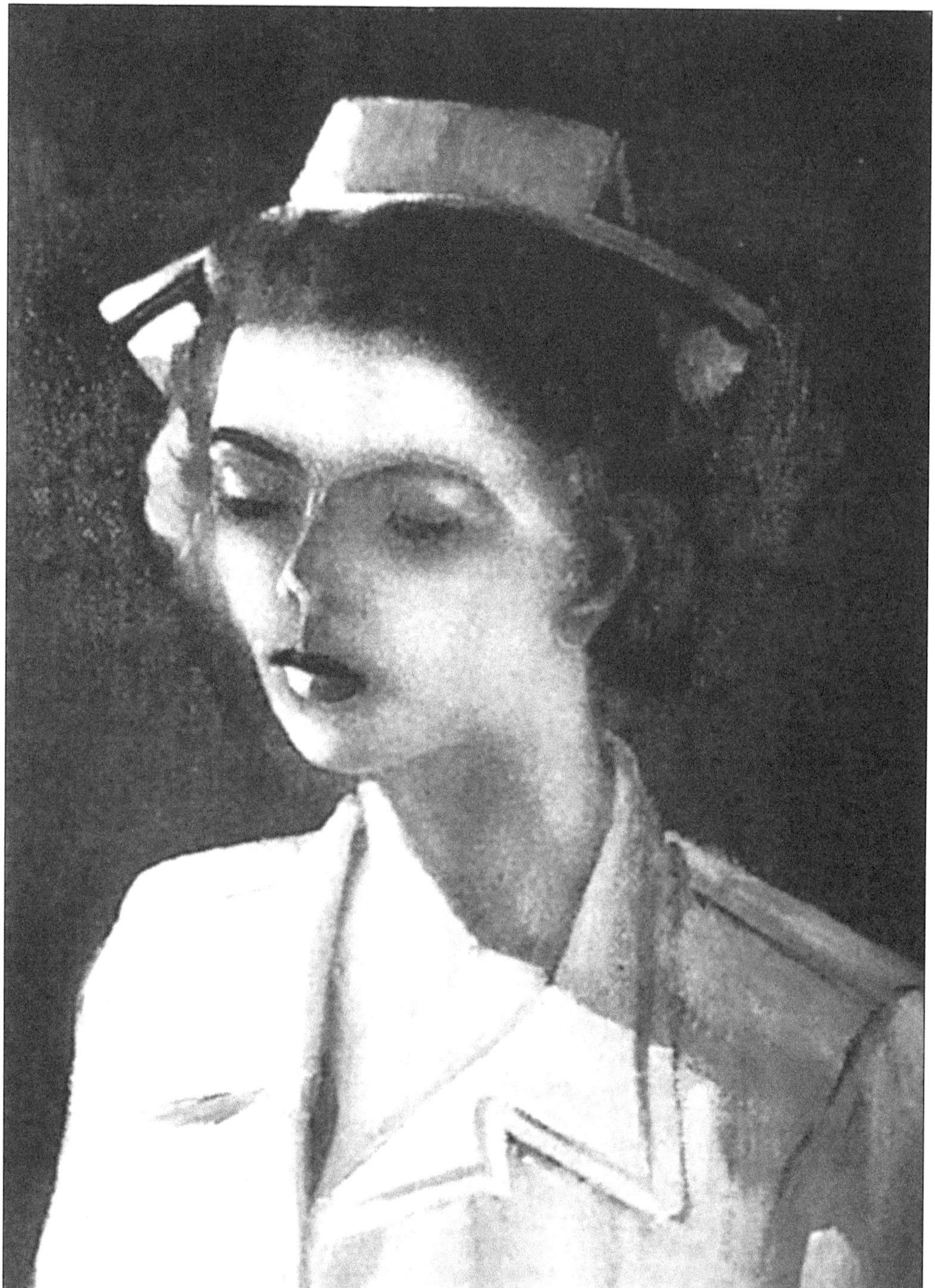

Richard Schmid, a young Chicago artist, water-colored his impression of a nurse standing in the shadow of the cross as his way of attracting attention to the Nurses Day special Novena service and parade in 1953. This was the cover of the *Novena Notes* one week prior to the event, which marked the fifth annual Nurses Day in Chicago as proclaimed by Governor Stratton and Chicago's Mayor Kennelly. (*Novena Notes*, May 15, 1953.)

Three

Twilight Spectacular
Nurses and Student Nurses Marching

"Two thousand uniformed nurses, their capes fluttering in the chill evening air, marched down Jackson Boulevard from Garfield Park last night in a colorful hour-long parade. The nurses were joined by 2,000 other marchers . . . from the Army, Navy, Marines, National Guard, and Chicago Police and Fire Departments. It was the 10th annual Nurses Day Parade." (*Chicago Daily Tribune*, May 10, 1958.)

All of the Nurses Day Parades were written about and photographed by Chicago newspapers, including the *Chicago Daily Tribune*, *Chicago Daily News*, *New World*, *Austin*, and the *Garfieldian*. Some parades even received national media coverage. One year the parade was filmed for a motion picture. Each year the parade had a different theme related to nursing or healthcare. A *New World* headline from May 20, 1955, said, "Nurses Day Parade Will Honor Discoverer of Polio Vaccine" and "Floats Depict Historic Find by Dr. Salk." Dr. Salk even wrote a letter stating why he could not attend this important parade honoring his discovery. Another theme honored student nurses, while another year focused on the diversity of nurses by highlighting nurses of different nationalities. A Native American nurse led the procession. A number of hospitals kept the theme of their float a secret, wanting to create excitement for the spectators and for the nurses. Often the most creative float was recognized and given an award. The parade was said to be as spectacular as any on Michigan Avenue. Nurses felt a sense of pride and had their "day of glory" as they passed the parade watchers, sometimes five- or six-people deep, cheering them on.

Father Brissette said, "Nurses who were accustomed to walking light-footed down dimly lighted corridors, marched with crisp step behind men swinging down the line to the rhythm of military music, passed spell-bound watchers and induced an electric excitement, and a rippling gasp of wonder."

The parade was meeting its goals of calling attention to the nurse shortage and honoring nurses. Perhaps it was a coincidence, but between 1949 to 1956, the enrollment in nursing schools had risen. It seems that the annual Nurses Day Parade had immeasurably aided the cause of nursing. Father Brissette hoped that after eight years, the Novena Service would go national. In the 10th year of the parade, no city had replicated Chicago's Nurses Day Parade. Nonetheless, the parade had a certain dramatic effect in calling attention to the unceasing need for more nurses. (John Long, *Novena Notes*, May 18, 1956, 11.)

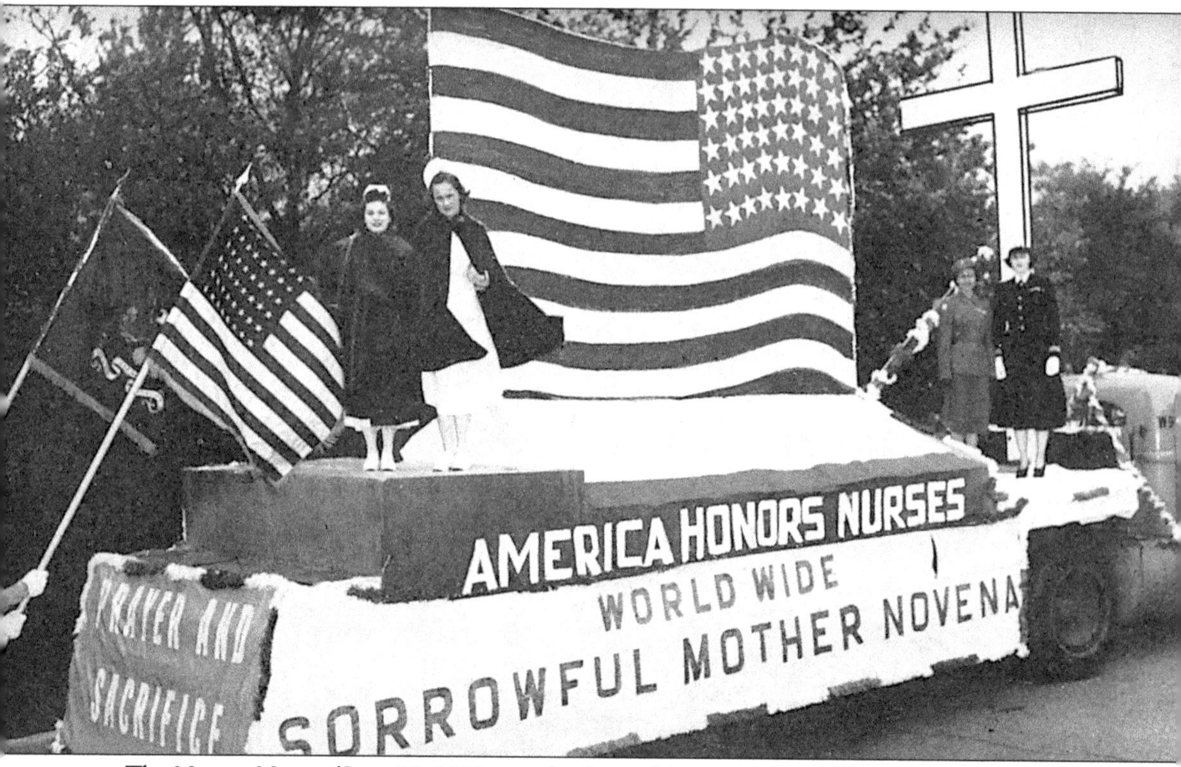

The *Novena Notes* of June 12, 1953, was the first publication of its kind in 16 years to devote the entire issue to photos. These photos were from the Nurses Day Parade, 1953. "One picture.... worth a thousand words. We are going to sit back and let our readers think." The cover of the *Novena Notes* was a float of America honoring nurses. The hope was that all nurses who left the National Shrine after the parade and service felt closer to the Mother of Sorrows regardless of their creed. (*Novena Notes*, June 12, 1953, cover.)

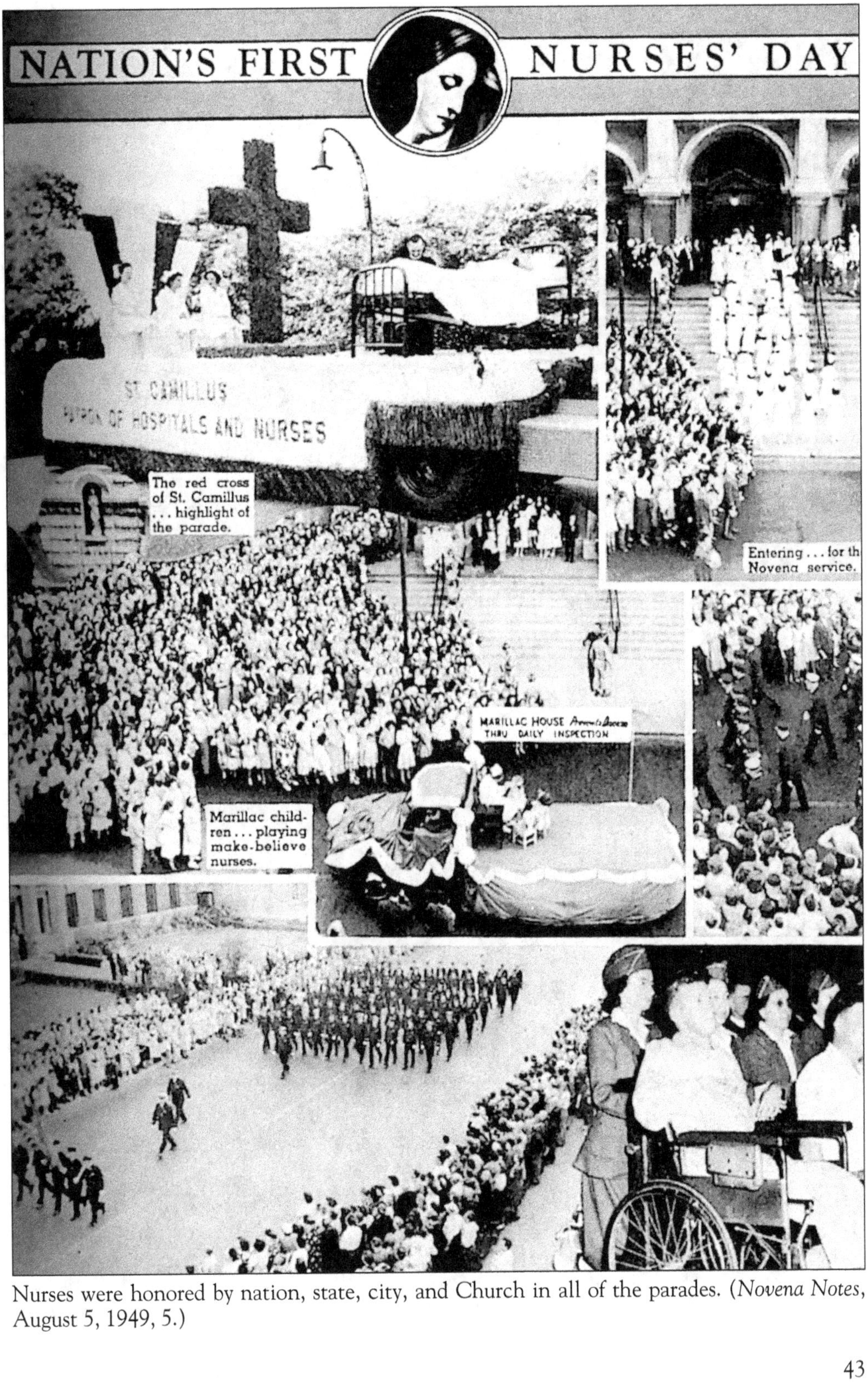
NATION'S FIRST NURSES' DAY
ST CAMILLUS
PATRON OF HOSPITALS AND NURSES
The red cross of St. Camillus . . . highlight of the parade.
Entering . . . for th Novena service.
MARILLAC HOUSE
THRU DAILY INSPECTION
Marillac children . . . playing make-believe nurses.

Nurses were honored by nation, state, city, and Church in all of the parades. (*Novena Notes*, August 5, 1949, 5.)

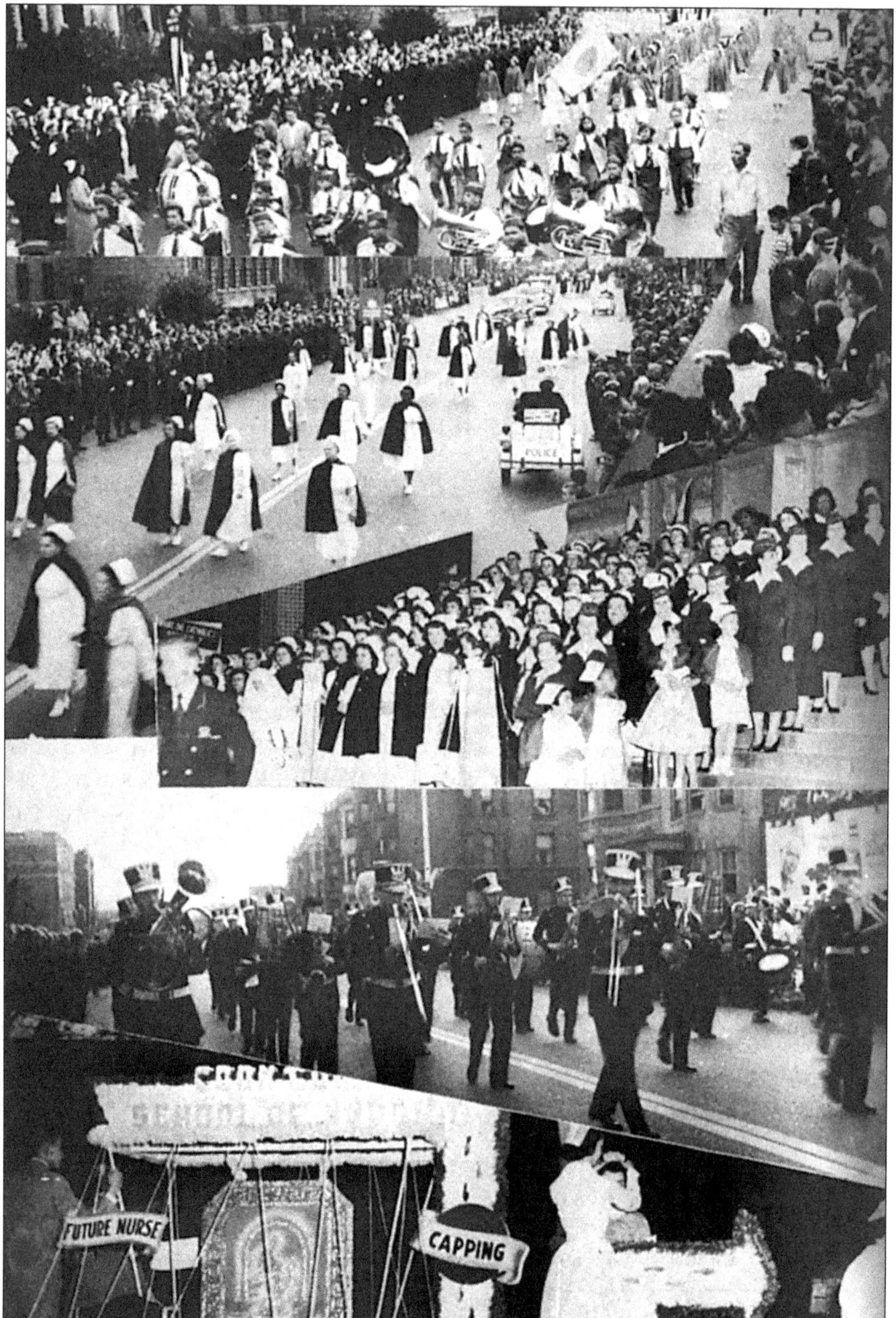

Cook County Hospital was the largest hospital in the nation in 1956. Their float illustrated a future nurse getting capped. (*Novena Notes*, June 8, 1956, 16.)

The sight of so many nurses marching with capes was astounding. (*Novena Notes*, June 10, 1955, 16.)

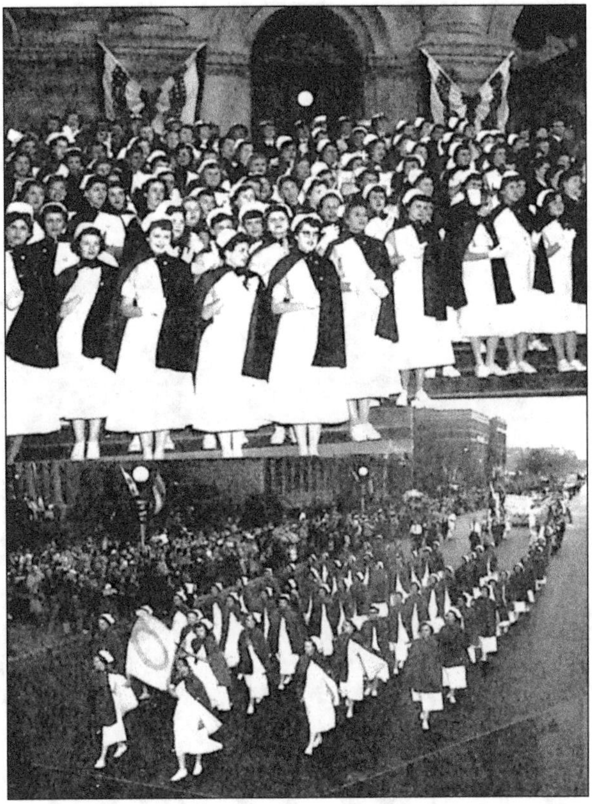

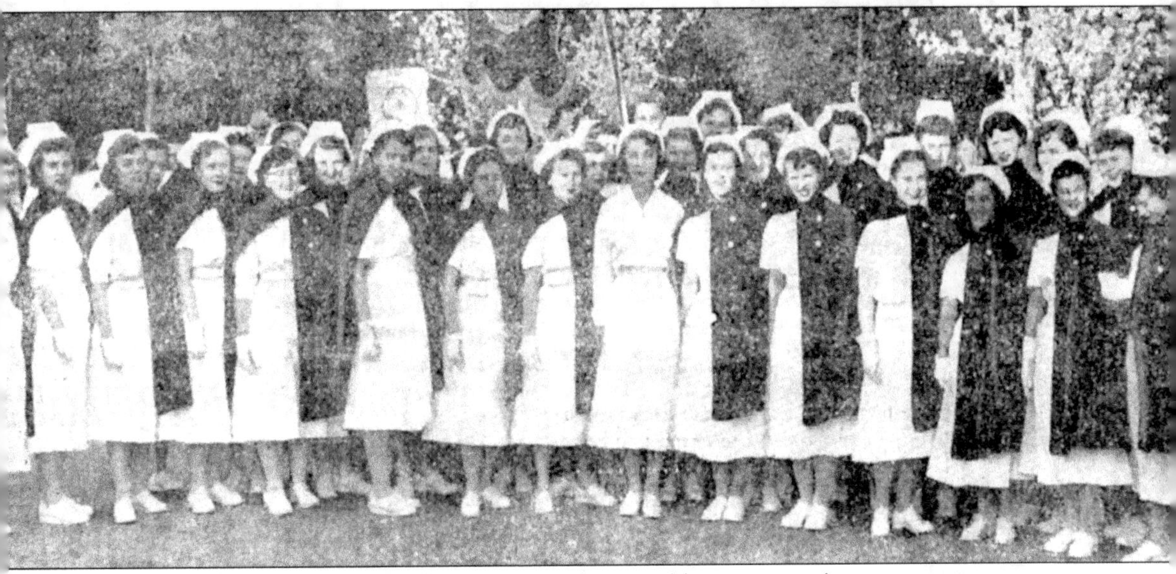

St. Joseph Hospital's nursing students are seen here in blue capes with a nursing instructor center stage. (*Chicago American Newspaper*.)

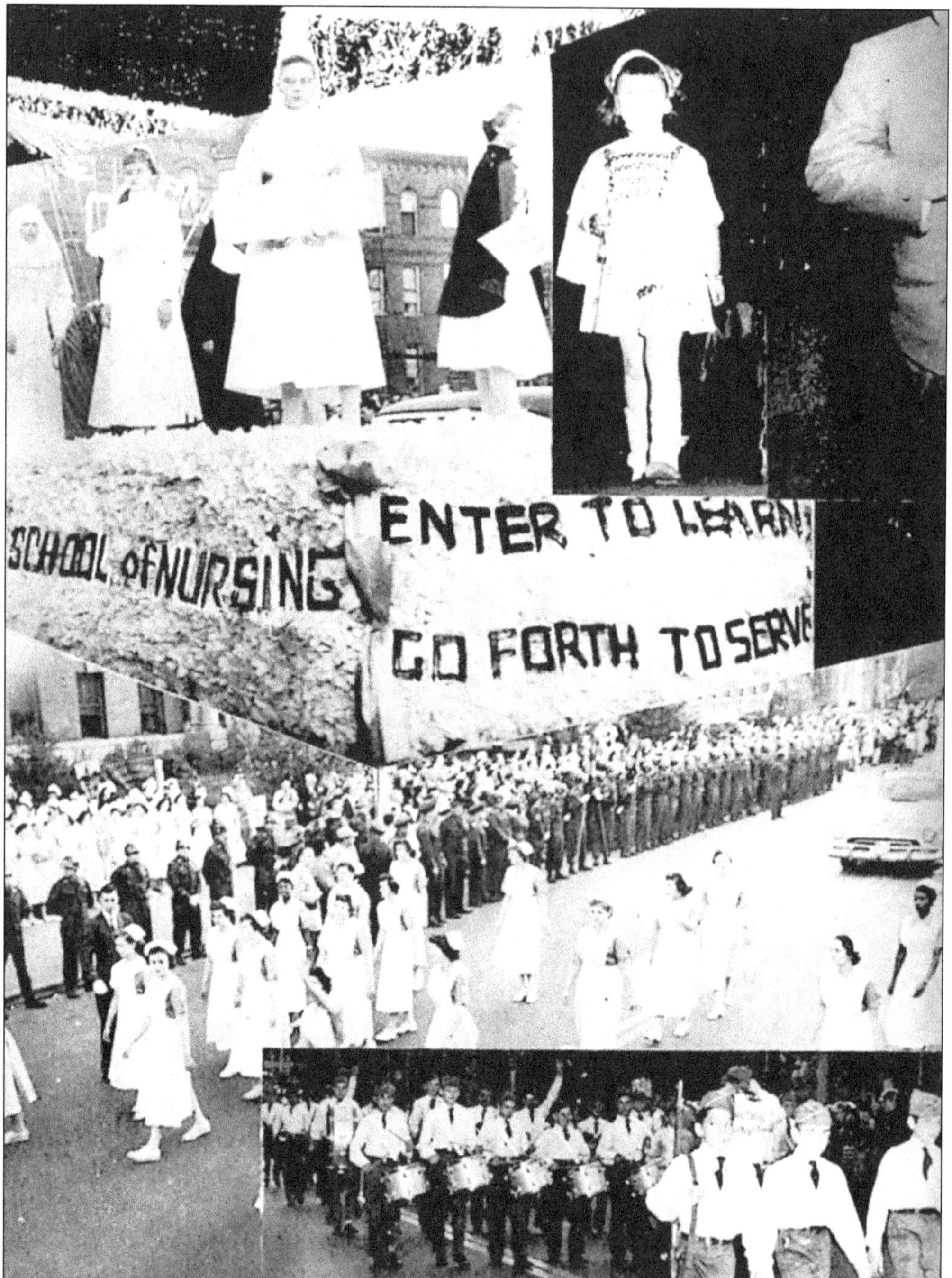
SCHOOL of NURSING
ENTER TO LEARN
GO FORTH TO SERVE
The recruitment of nurses into the profession was a goal of the parade. The majority of the Chicagoland schools of nursing marched in the parade. (*Novena Notes*, June 8, 1956, 14.)

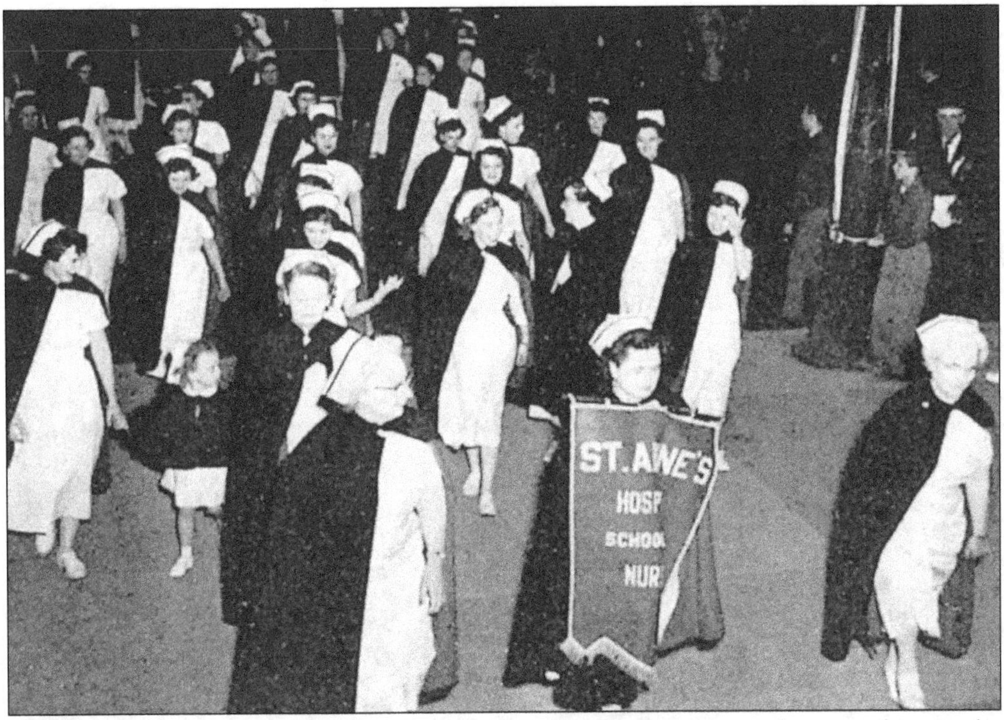

St. Anne's Hospital School of Nursing students and instructors are seen here marching in the 1954 parade. (*Novena Notes*, June 11, 1954, 5.)

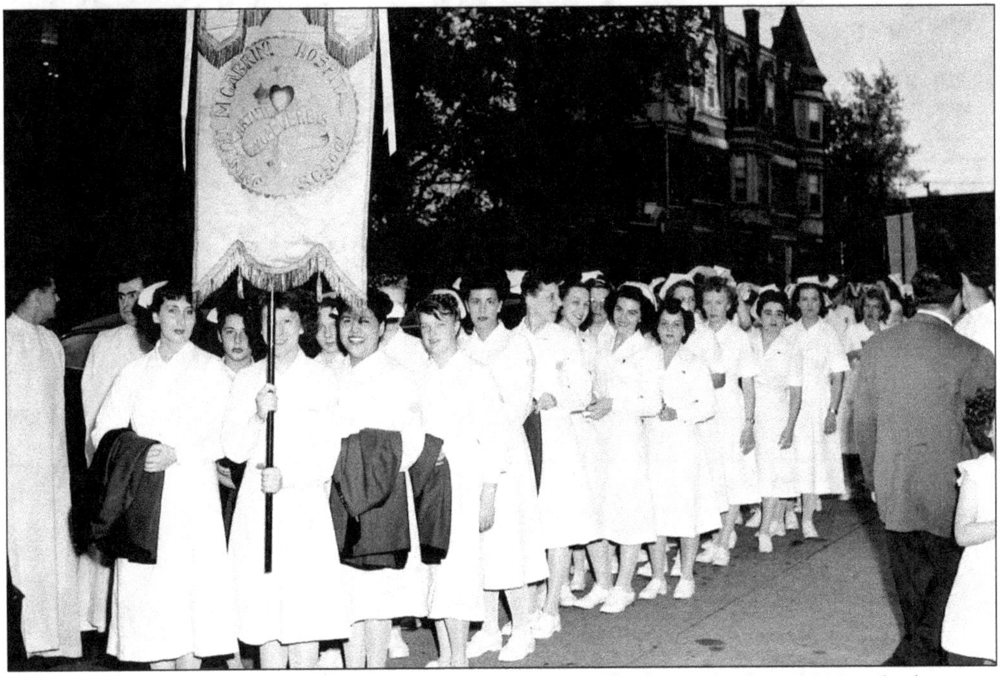

Nurses and students from Cabrini Hospital Nursing School marched in 1948, which was a prelude to the first Nurses Day Parade in 1949. (This photo also appeared in the *Novena Notes*, August 6, 1948, 8–9.)

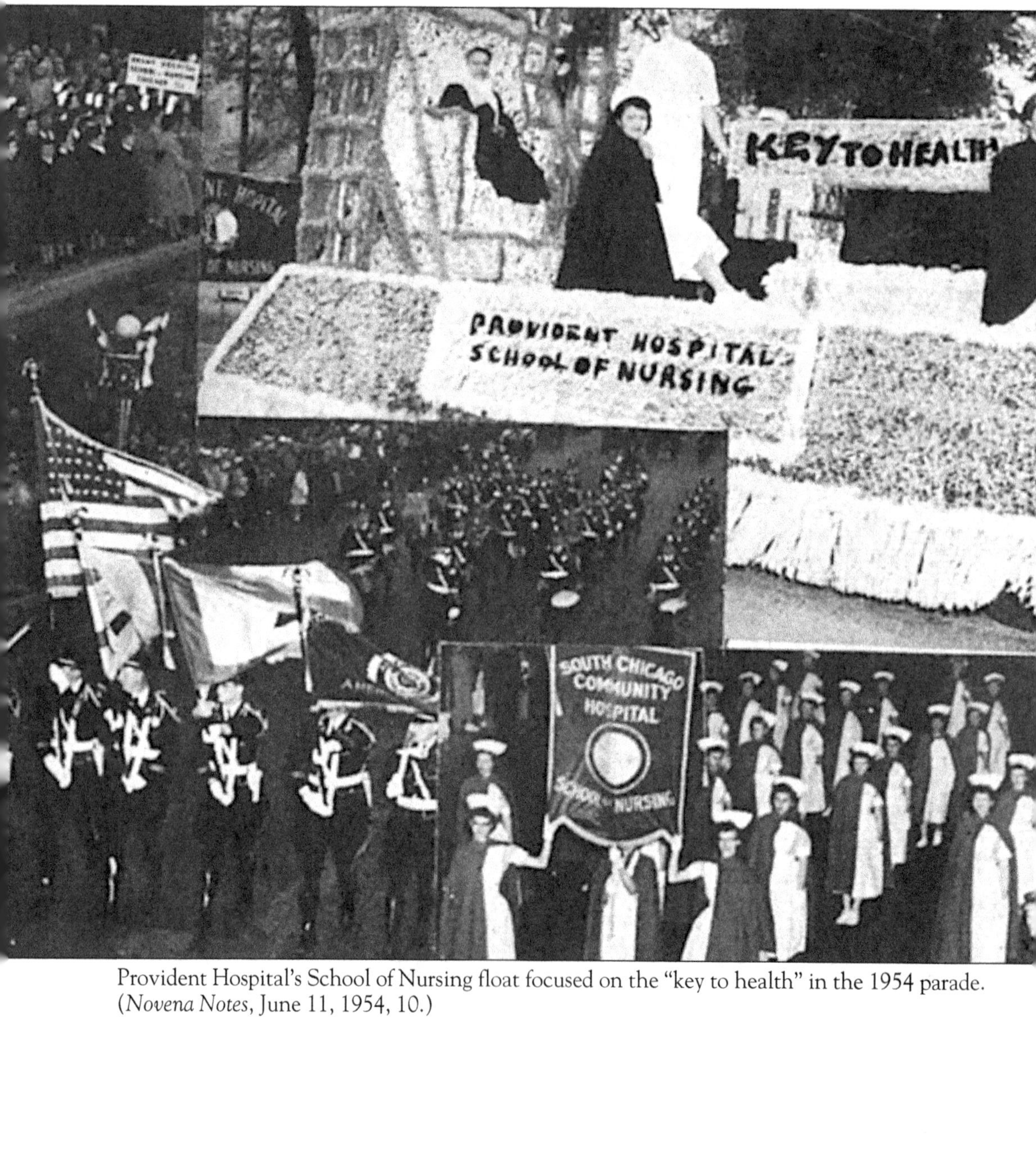

Provident Hospital's School of Nursing float focused on the "key to health" in the 1954 parade. (*Novena Notes*, June 11, 1954, 10.)

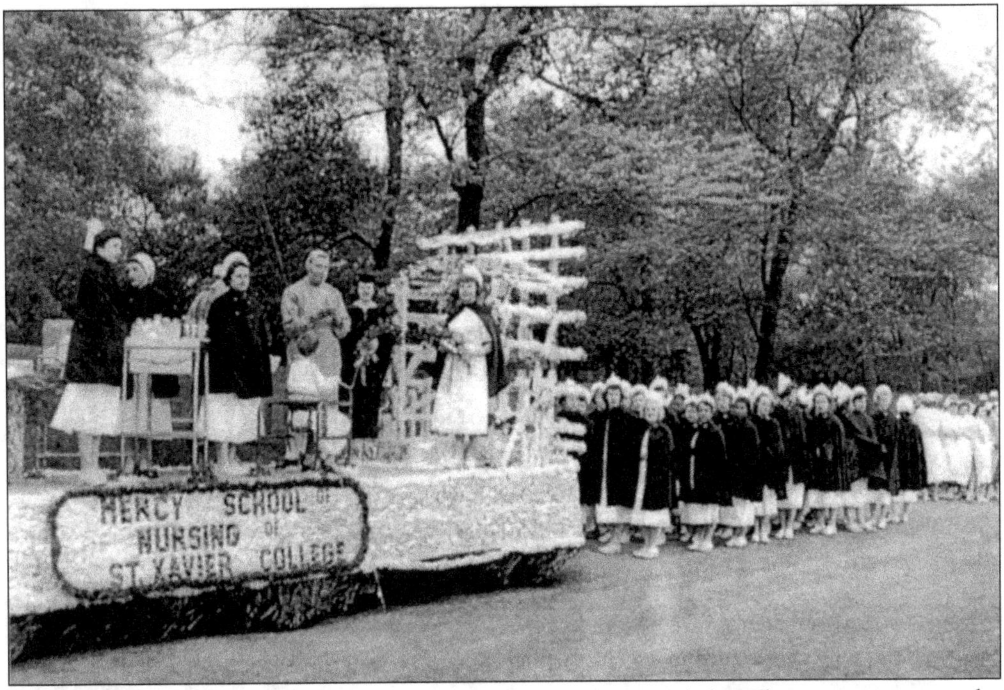

The 10th annual Nurses Day Parade was called a spectator's delight. The spectators were the most demonstrative of all parade audiences, calling out and cheering nurses as they passed in the parade. No one imagined at that time that this would be the last Nurses Day Parade. (*Novena Notes*, May 30th, 1958, 13.) (Photo permission from Mercy Hospital.)

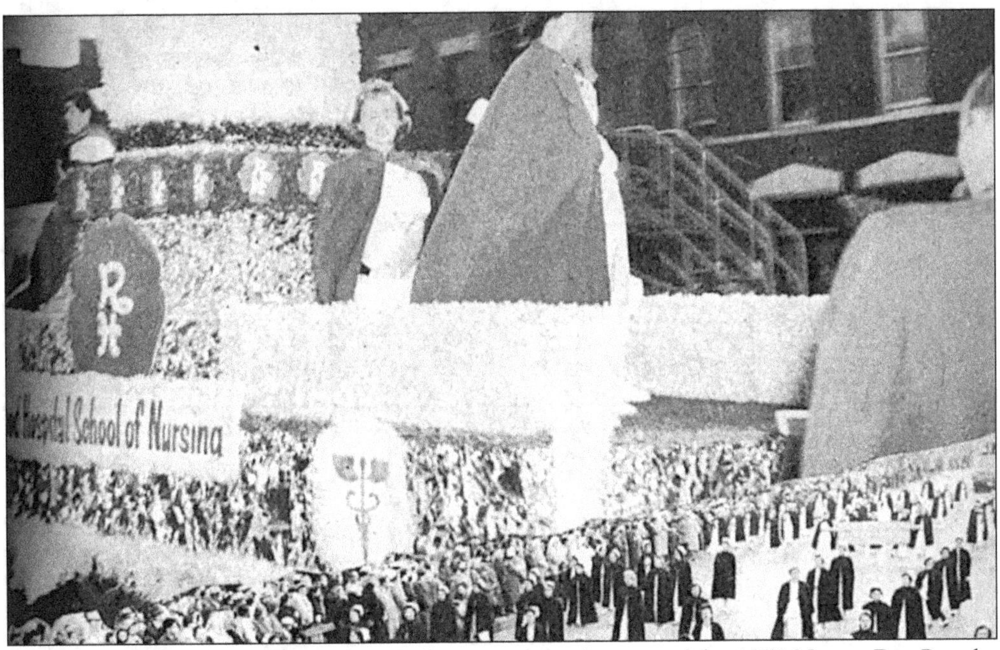

Ravenswood Hospital celebrated its 60th anniversary the year of the 1958 Nurses Day Parade. (*Novena Notes*, May 30, 1958, 3.)

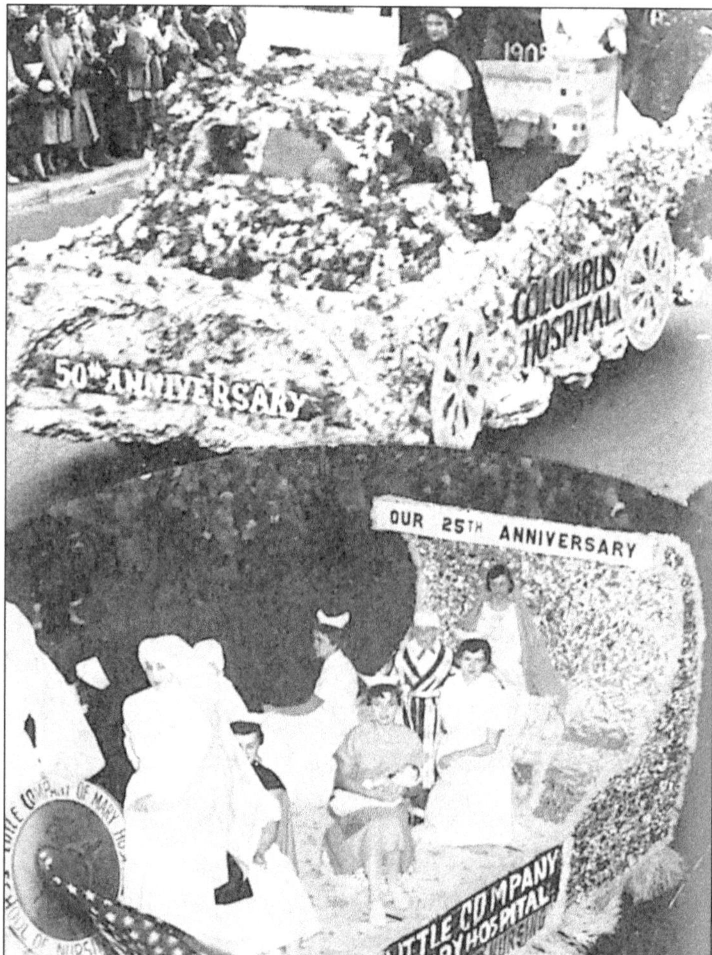

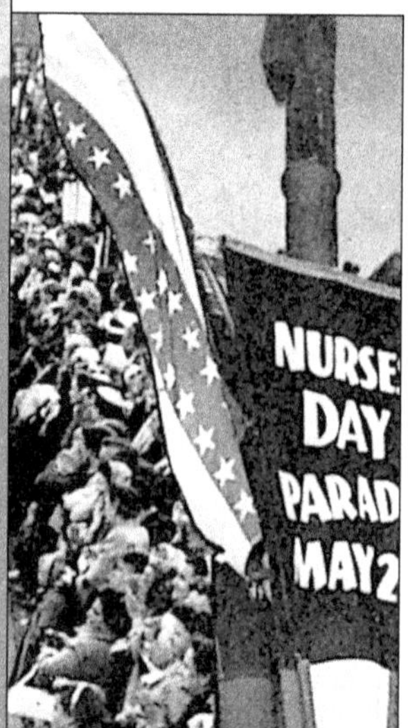

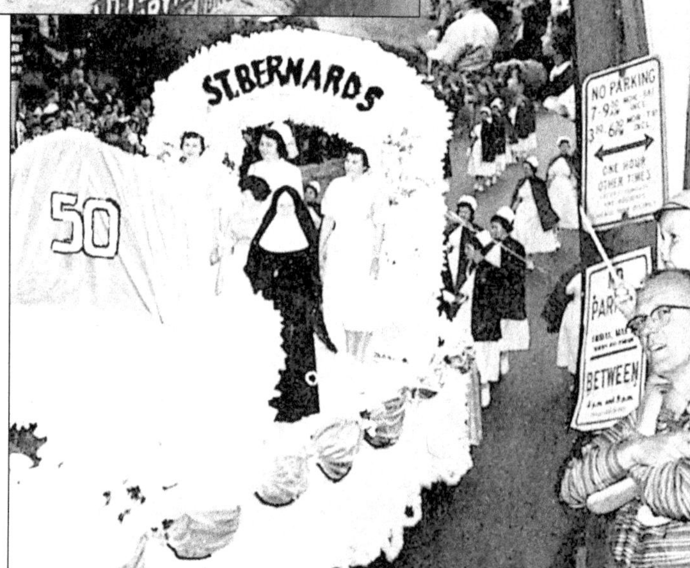

The year 1955 marked the 50th anniversary of Columbus and St. Bernard's Hospitals and the 25th anniversary of the Little Company of Mary Hospital. All celebrated with floats in the Nurses Day Parade. (*Novena Notes*, June 10, 1955, 8–9.)

The year 1957 marked the 50th anniversary of Oak Park Hospital, so its float and marchers were placed up front in the 1957 parade. (John Long, *Novena Notes* May 31, 1957, 8.)

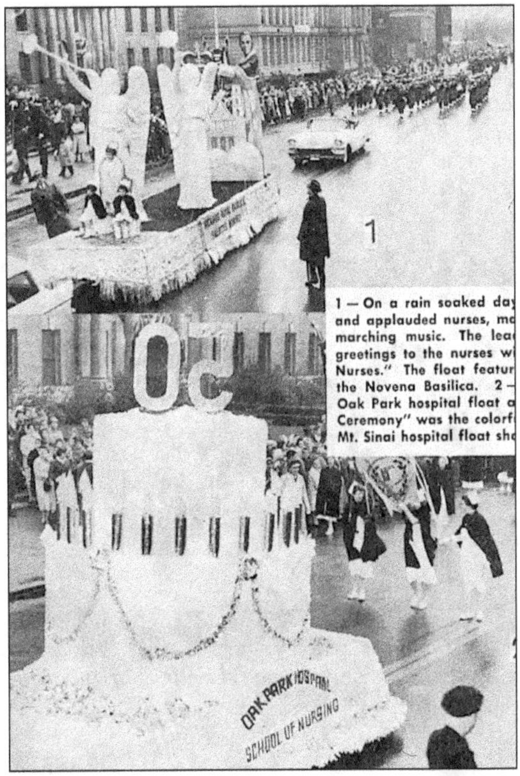
1
1 — On a rain soaked da
and applauded nurses, m
marching music. The lea
greetings to the nurses w
Nurses." The float featur
the Novena Basilica. 2 –
Oak Park hospital float a
Ceremony" was the colorf
Mt. Sinai hospital float sh
50
OAK PARK HOSPITAL
SCHOOL OF NURSING

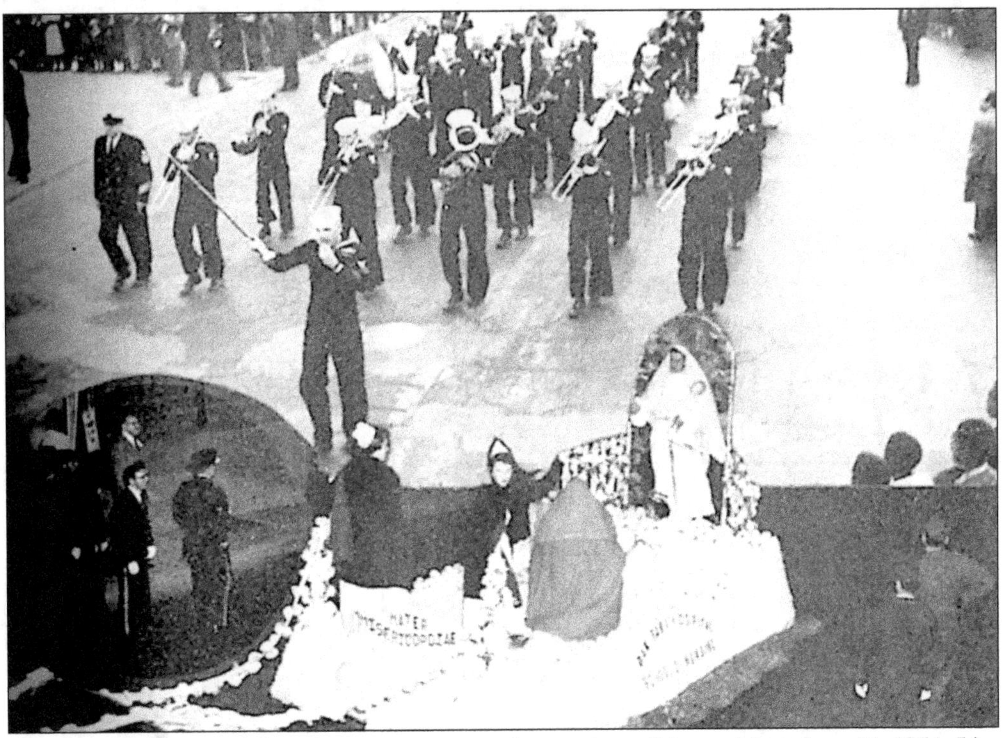

This Oak Park Hospital float shows nurses caring for a patient. (*Novena Notes*, June 11, 1954, 5.)

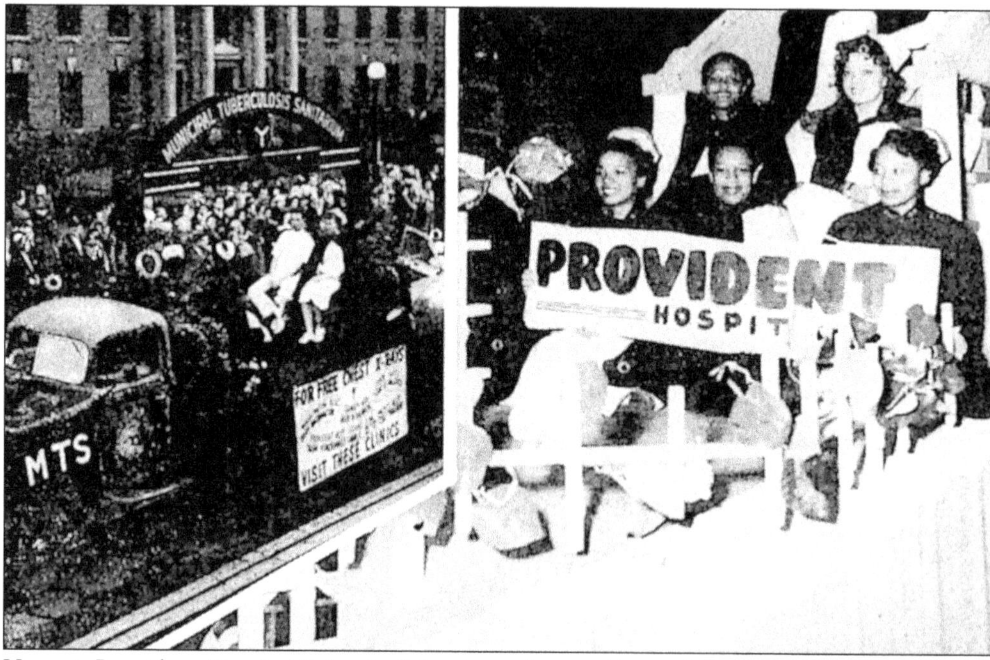

Historic Provident Hospital School of Nursing is featured here. (*Novena Notes*, June 13, 1952, 16.)

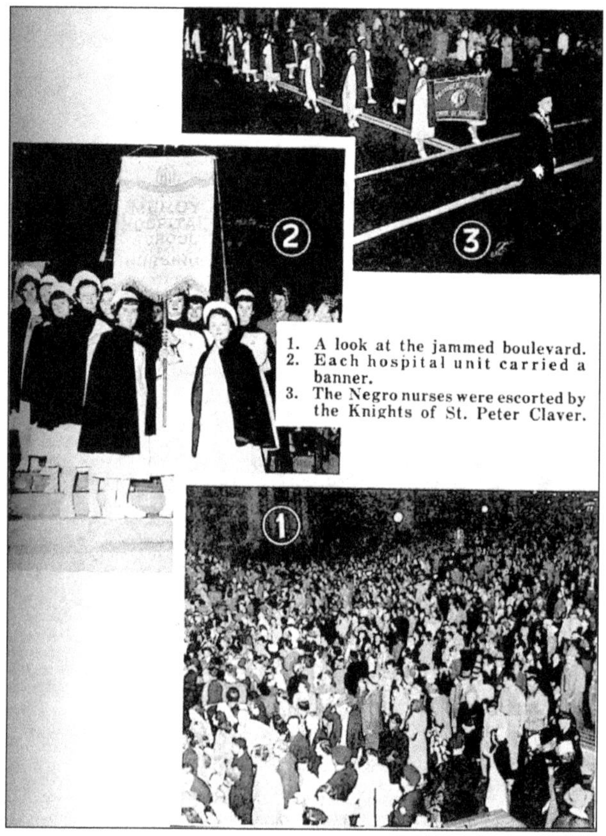
1. A look at the jammed boulevard.
2. Each hospital unit carried a banner.
3. The Negro nurses were escorted by the Knights of St. Peter Claver.

Nurses truly enjoyed their "day of glory," as seen in the 1950 Nurses Day Parade. (*Novena Notes*, October 6, 1950, 13.)

Marchers are seen here honoring nurses in the 1953 parade. (*Novena Notes*, June 12, 1953, 6.)

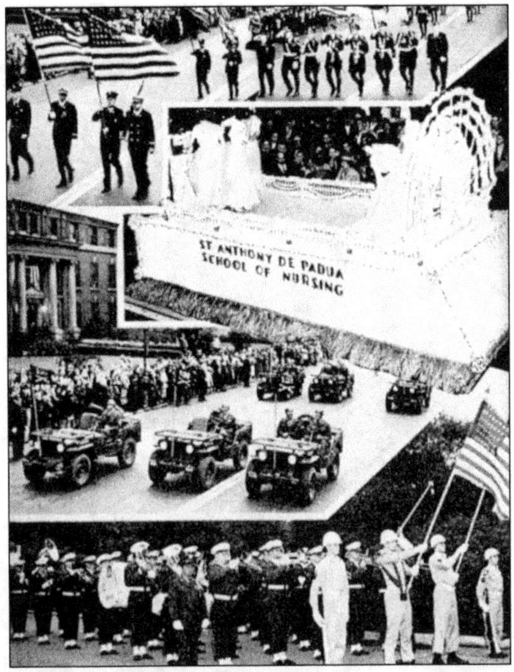

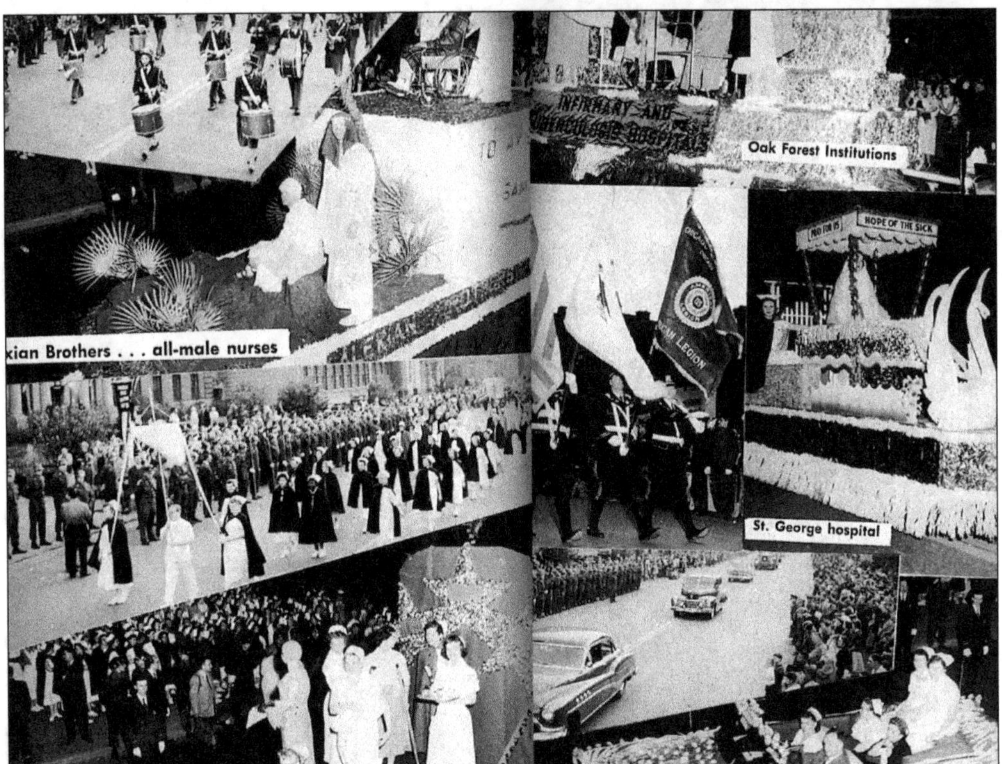

These are scenes from the 1956 Nurses Day Parade in which Father Brissette pointed out that the distance of the march for the nurses was kept purposefully short in deference to the nurses who daily piled up mileage in hospital corridors. (*Novena Notes*, June 8, 1956, 10–11.)

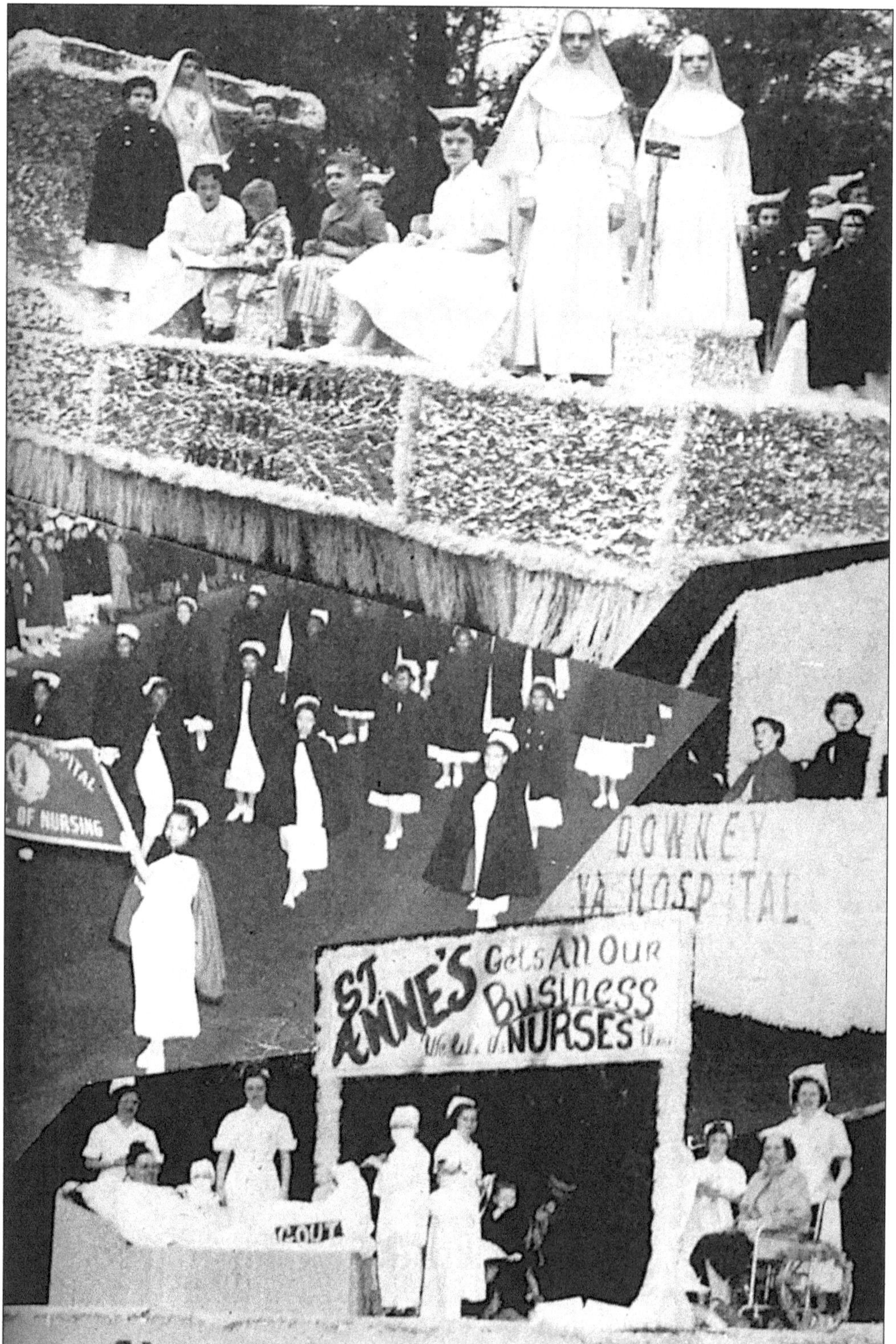

St. Anne's float depicts a nurse caring for a patient with gout. (*Novena Notes*, June 11, 1954, 11.)

Previous Nurses Day Parade highlights were featured on the cover of the *Novena Notes* on May 9th, 1958, the date of the last parade.

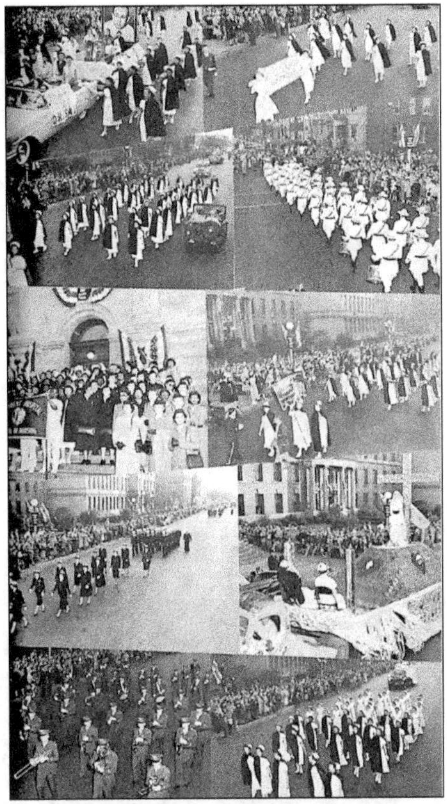

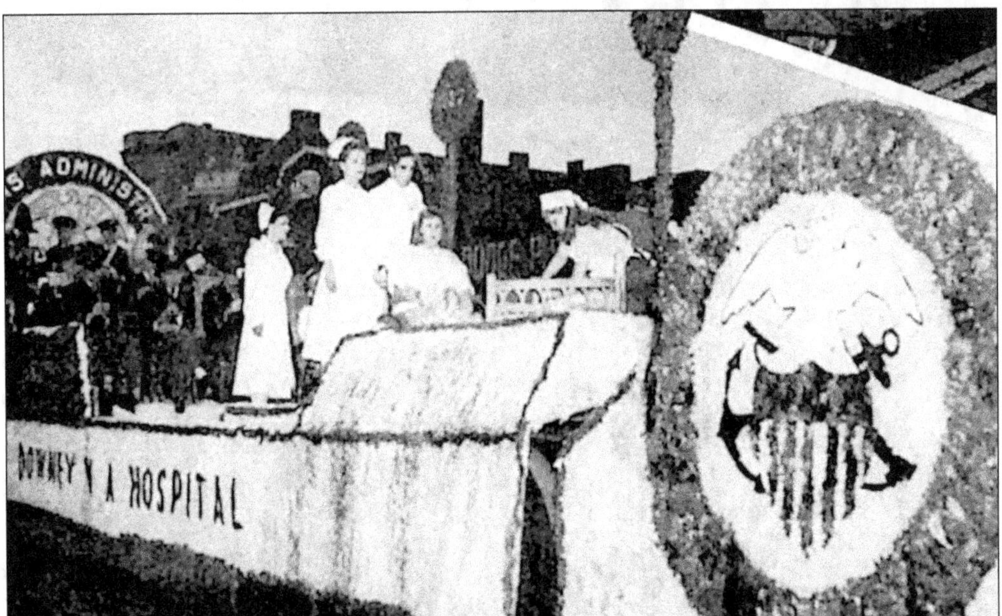

The Veterans Administration Hospital's decorative float is seen here. (*Novena Notes*, June 13, 1952, 4.)

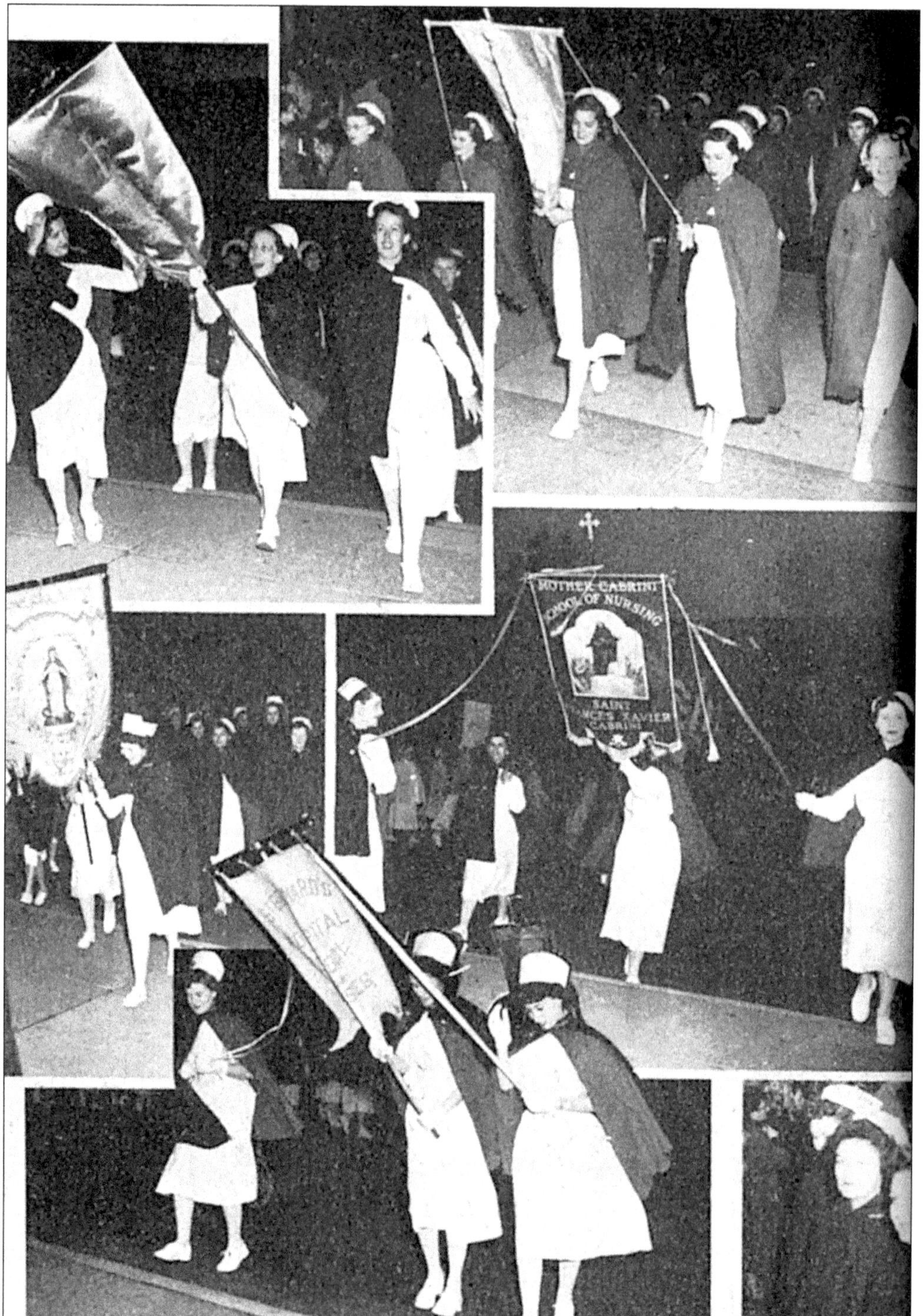

Nurses with banners and smiles took a brisk "right about turn into the wind" during the 1953 Nurses Day Parade. (*Novena Notes*, June 12, 1953, 14.)

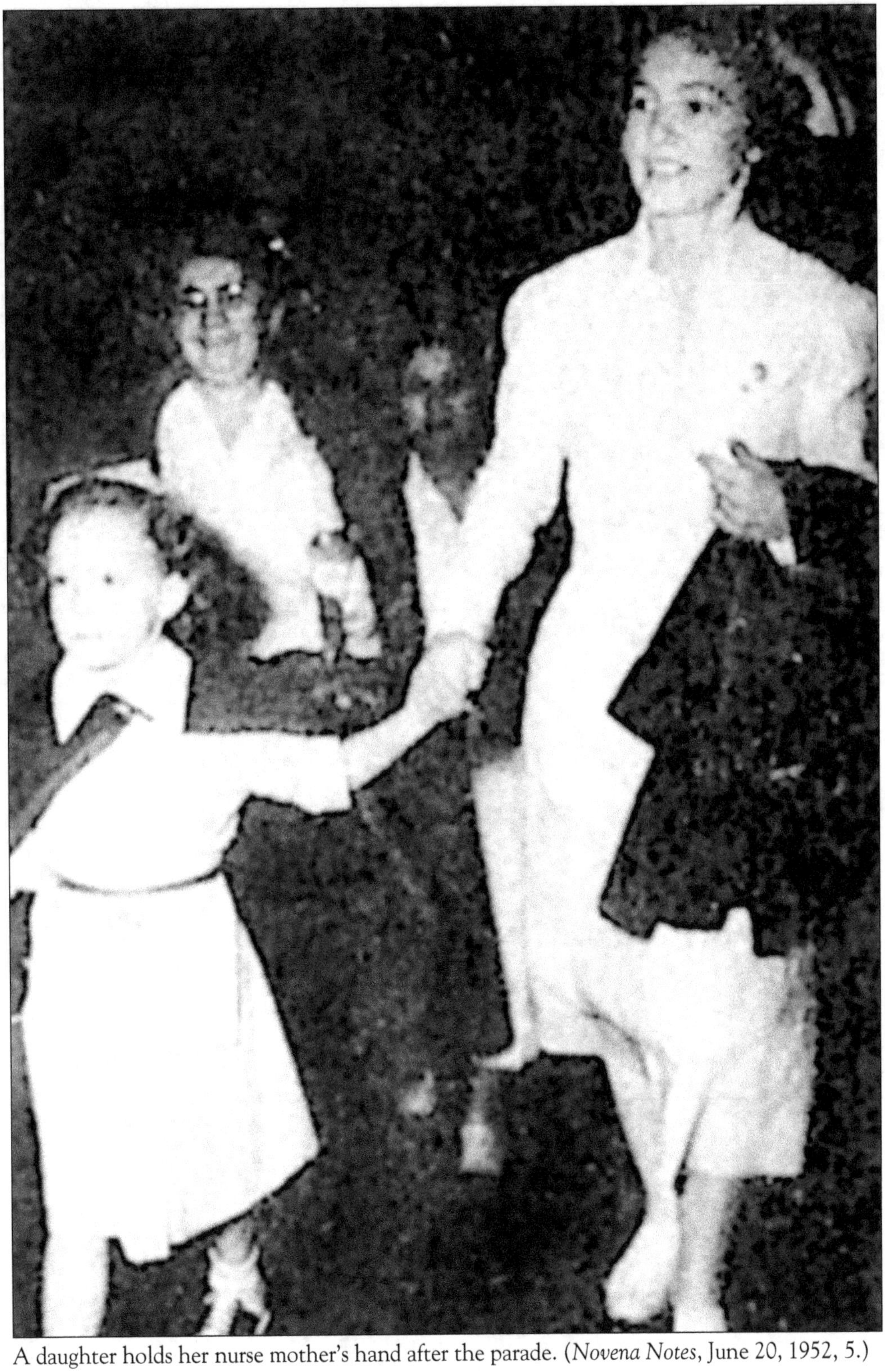

A daughter holds her nurse mother's hand after the parade. (*Novena Notes*, June 20, 1952, 5.)

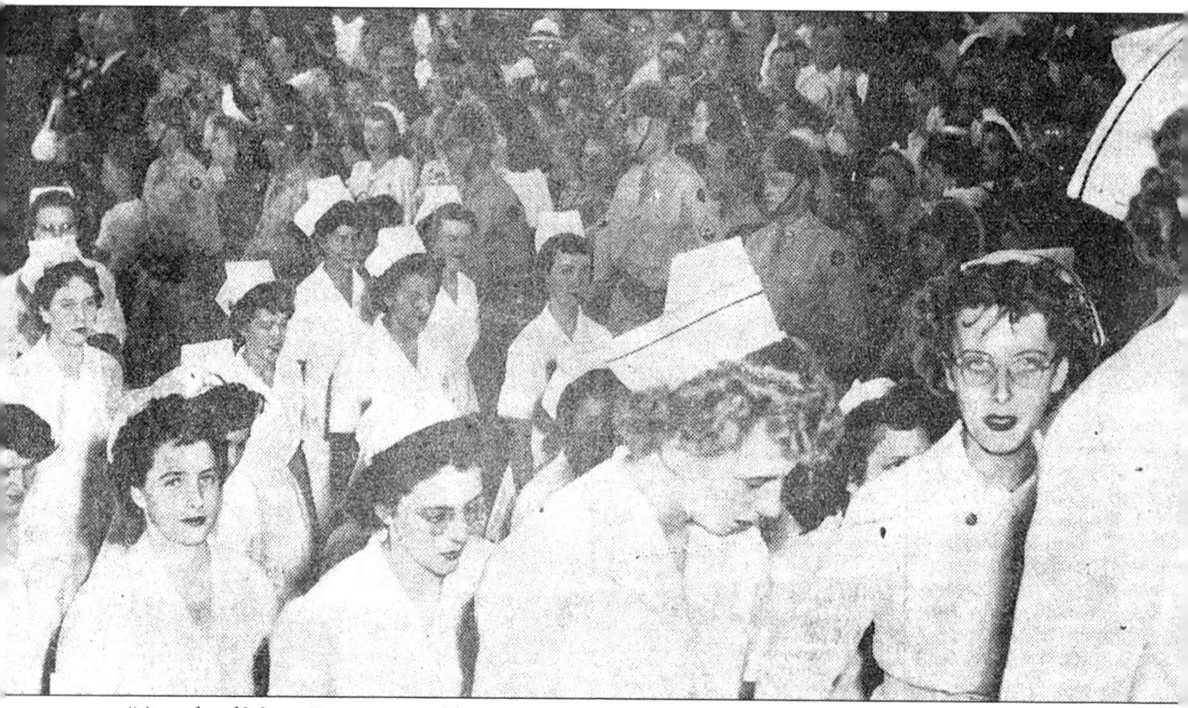

"Angels of Mercy" are pictured here entering Our Lady of Sorrows Basilica after the parade.

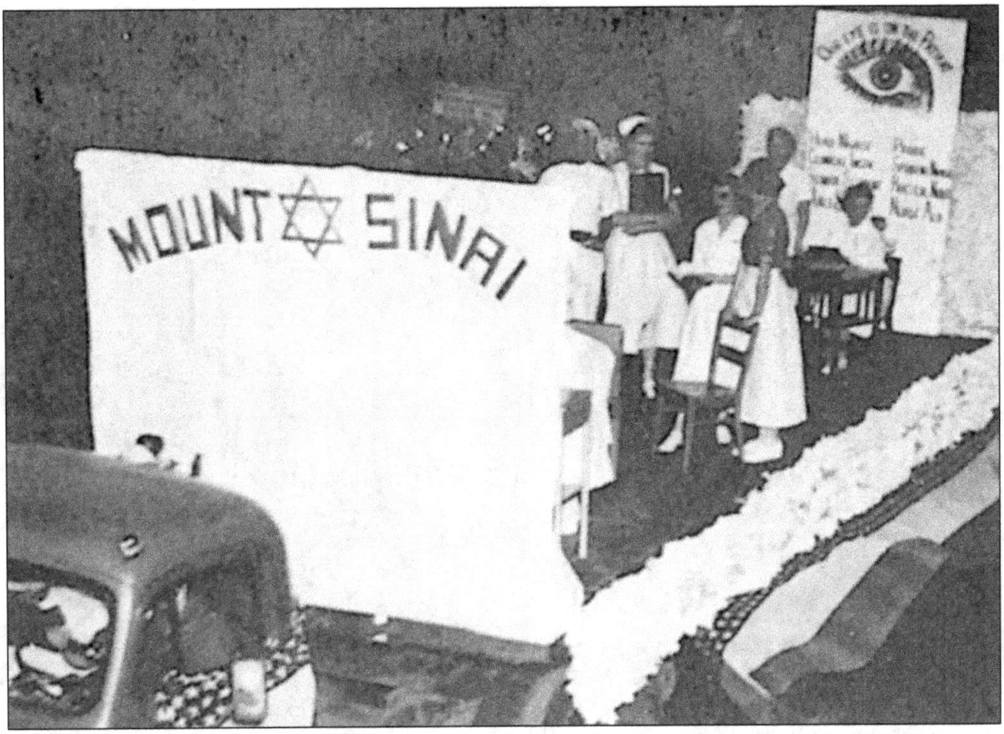

The Star of David was featured on Mount Sinai's float. (*Novena Notes*, June 11, 1954, 4.)

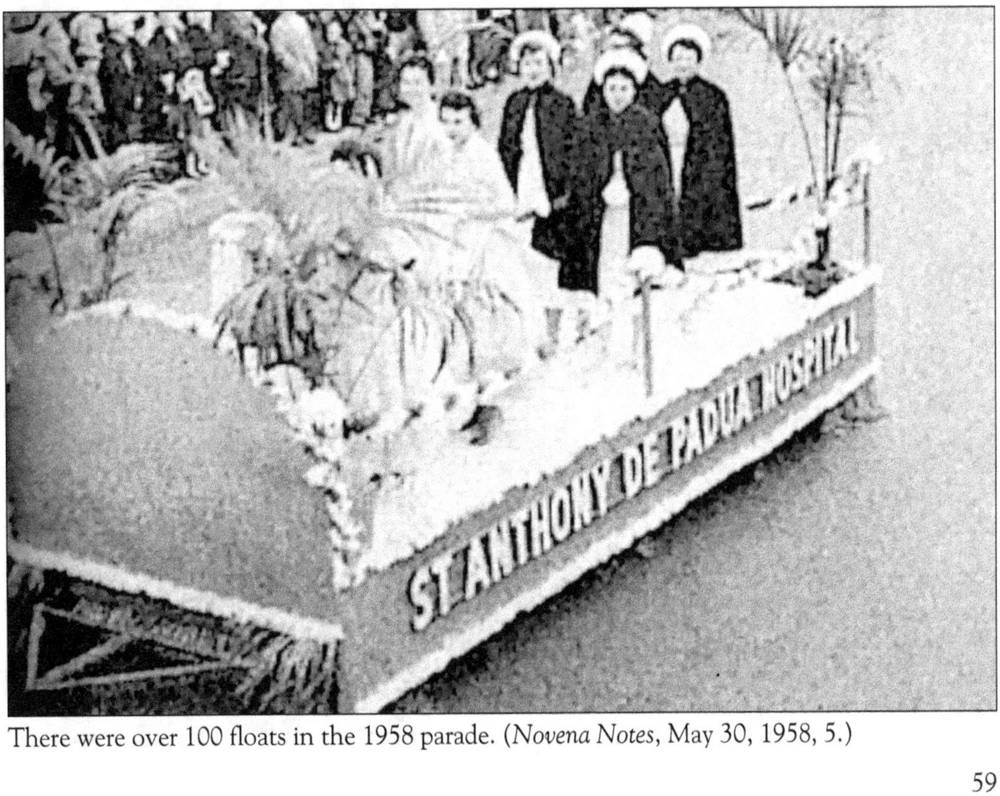

There were over 100 floats in the 1958 parade. (*Novena Notes*, May 30, 1958, 5.)

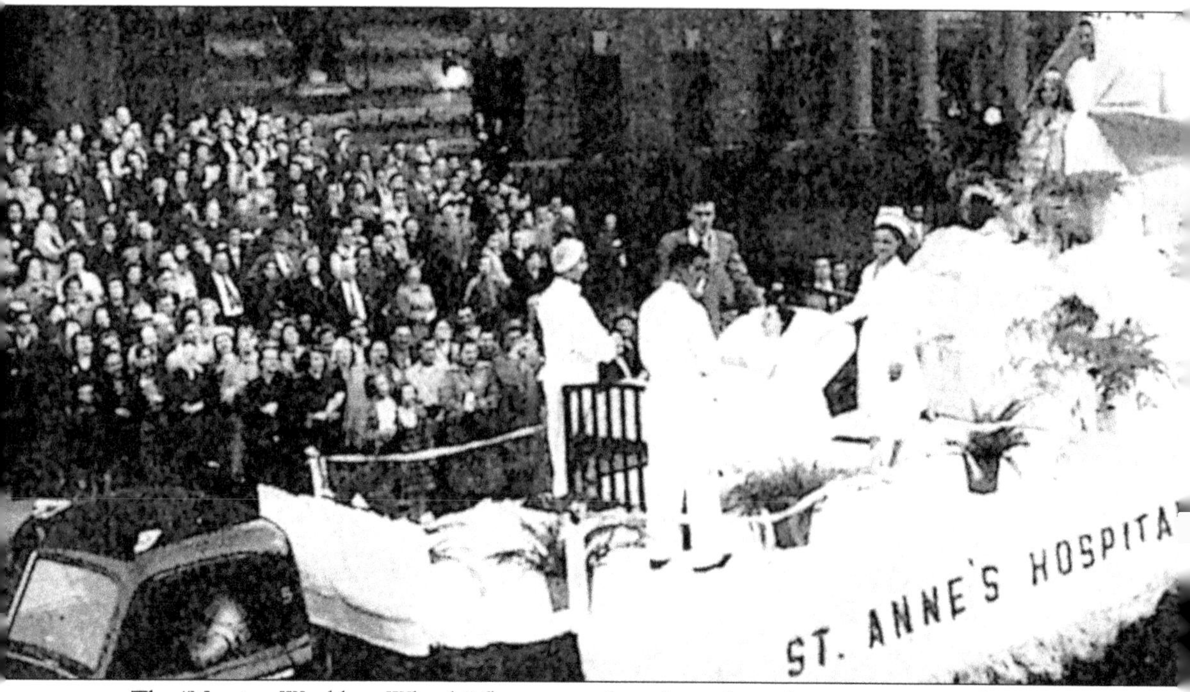

The "Nursing World on Wheels" floats contributed greatly to the excitement and pageantry in the 1952 parade. (*Novena Notes*, June 13, 1952, 5.)

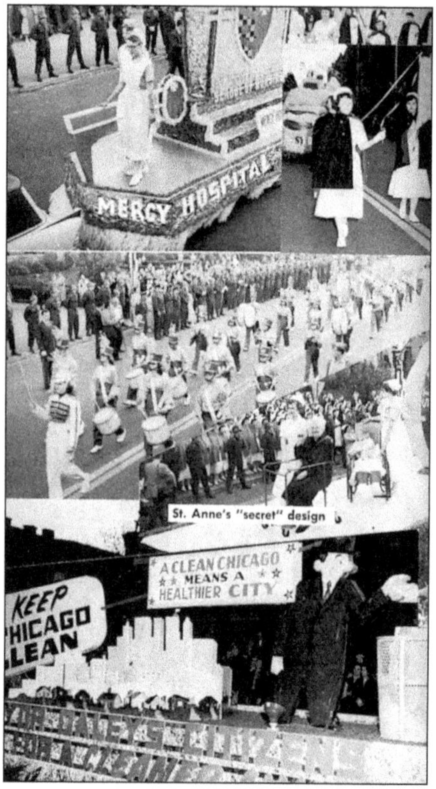

Many times the themes of the floats were kept a secret to surprise the spectators and create excitement. St. Anne's had a "secret" design. (*Novena Notes*, June 8, 1956, 6.)

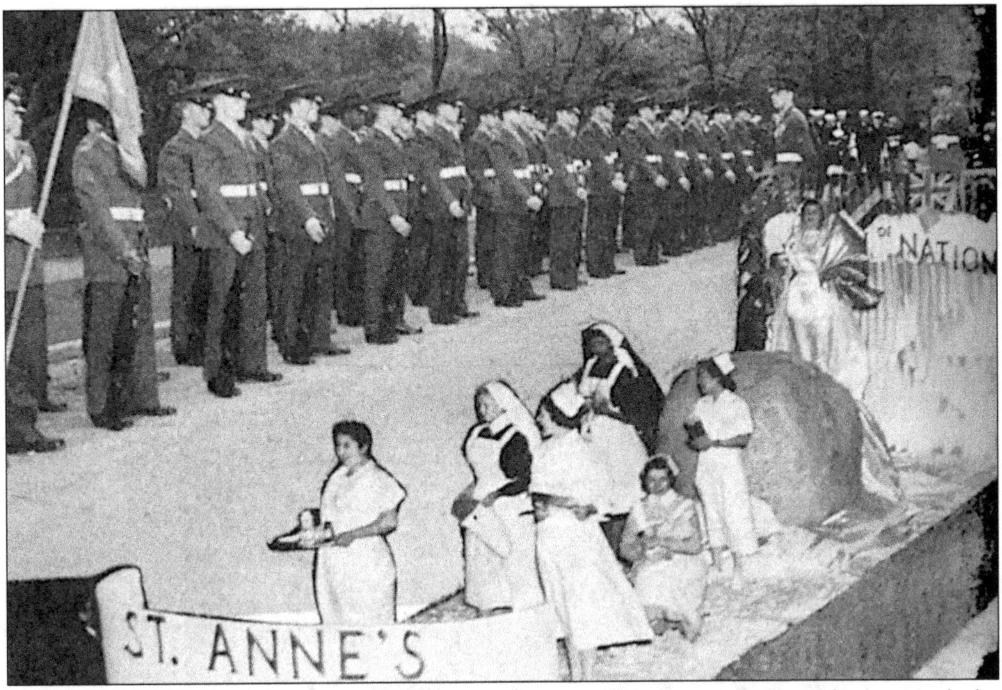

In 1954, the floats told of the work of nurses. Resurrection was the newest Chicago Catholic Hospital. Though they were not expected to have a float due to the newness of their hospital, they did have one, and set the standard high for the next year's parade. Above is a float designed by St. Anne's Hospital. (*Novena Notes*, June 11, 1954, 14.)

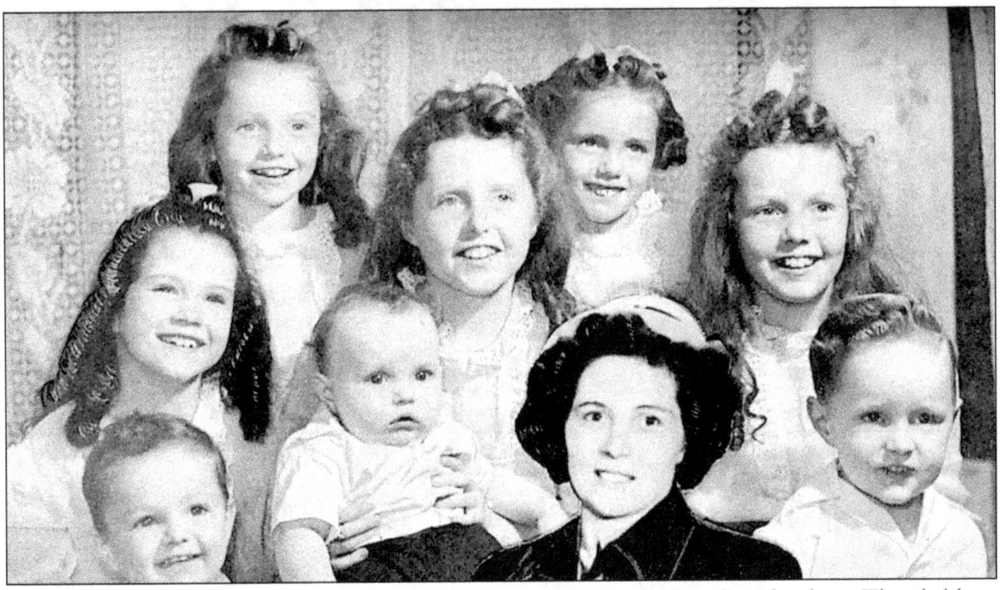

The Brennan family was very secretive about their 1955 Nurses Day Parade plans. The children ranged in age from 2 to 15 years old and were having difficulty keeping their lips sealed. "All we'll say is that we'll be in the parade with a float." The children kept close guard on their garage to protect their secret. All thirteen of the Brennan children were born at St. Anne's Hospital. (Tom Seery, *Novena Notes*, 1955, Picture from *Novena Notes*, May 12, 1950, cover.)

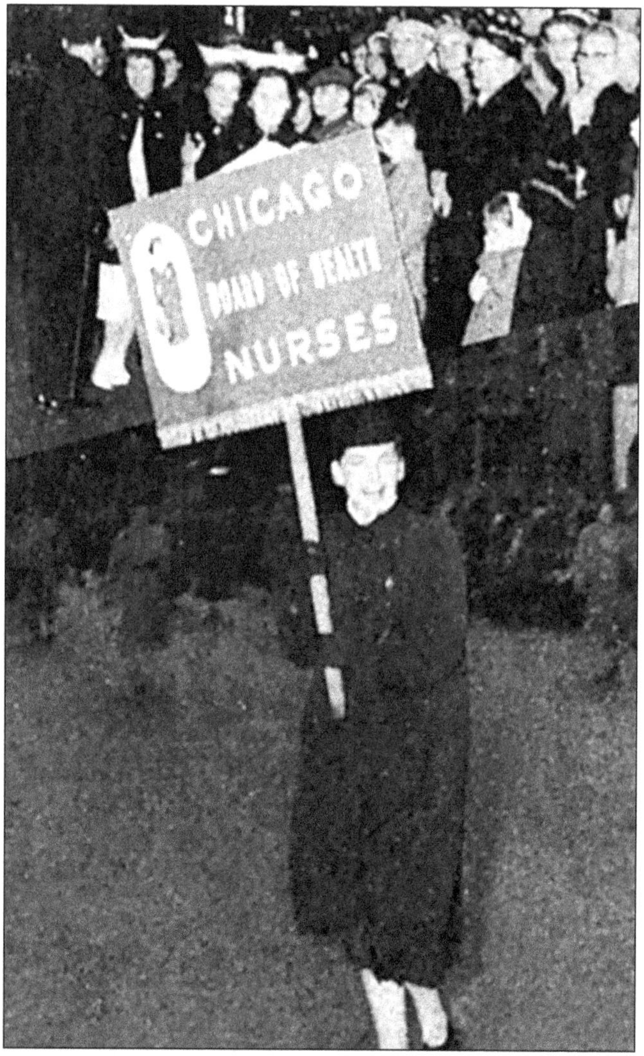

The Chicago Board of Health nurses also marched in the 1958 parade. (*Novena Notes*, May 30, 1958, 15.)

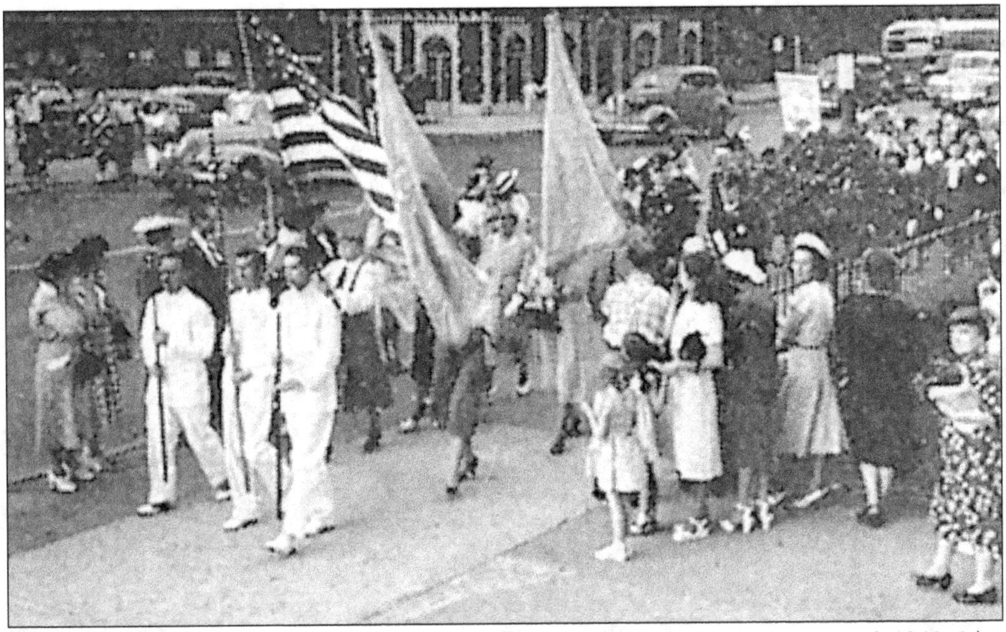

Male nurses marched in the prelude to the parade in 1948. (*Novena Notes*, August 6, 1948, 8.)

"Angels of Mercy" gathered in the Basilica to renew their nurse's pledge after parade. (*Novena Notes*, October 6, 1950, 5.)

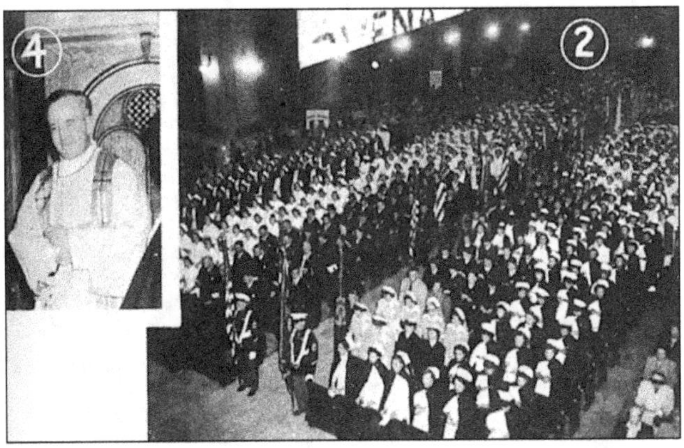

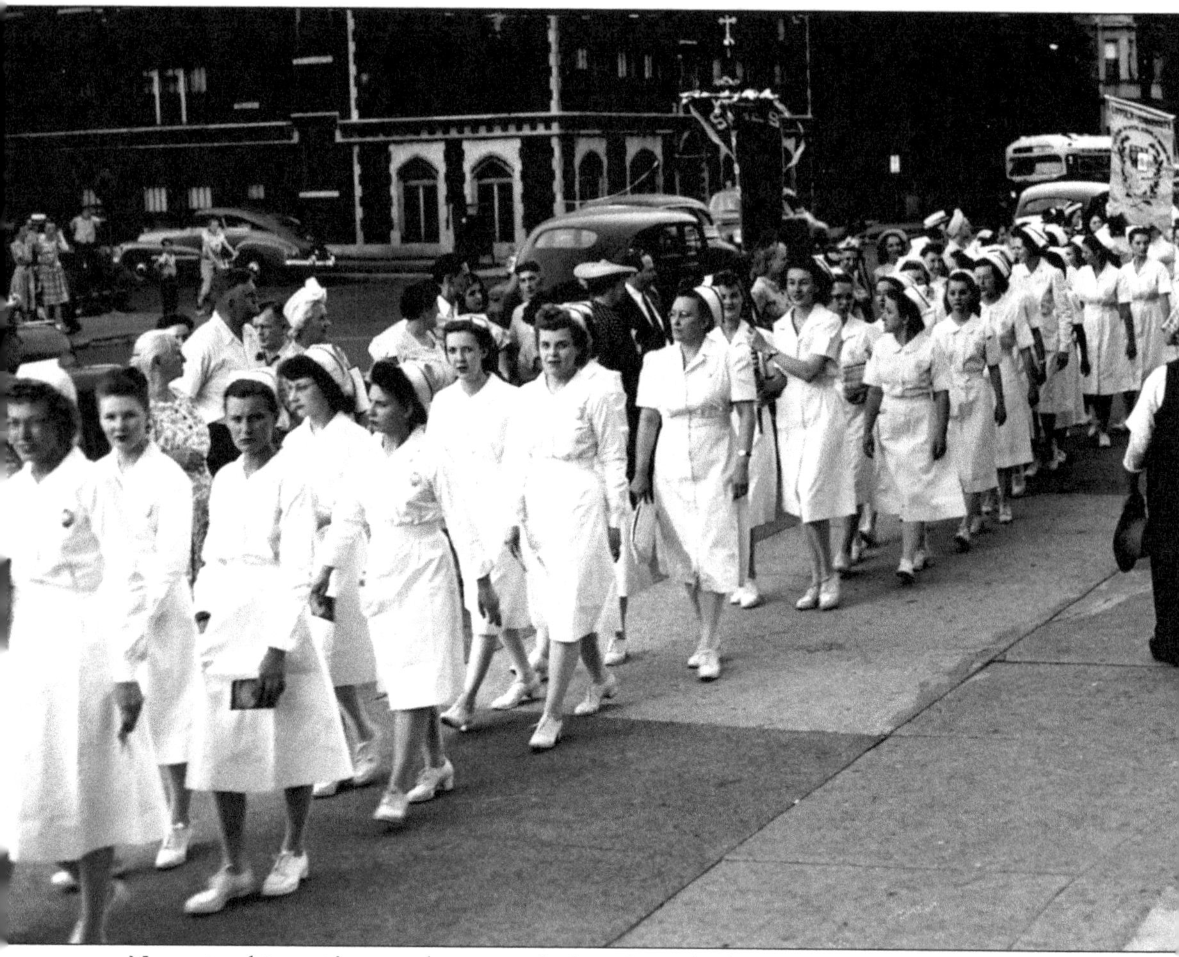

Nurses in white uniforms and caps marched in 1948, which was a prelude to the first Nurses Day Parade in 1949. (This photo appeared in the *Novena Notes*, August 6, 1948, 8.)

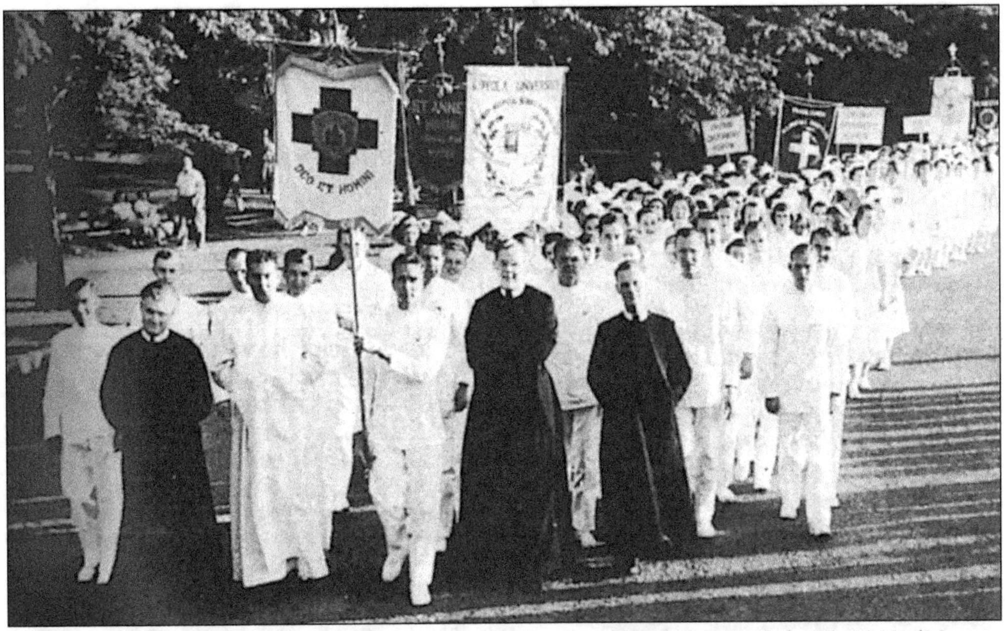

Alexian Brothers Hospital's male nurses are seen leading the parade on July 15, 1949. (*Novena Notes*, August 5, 1949, 11.)

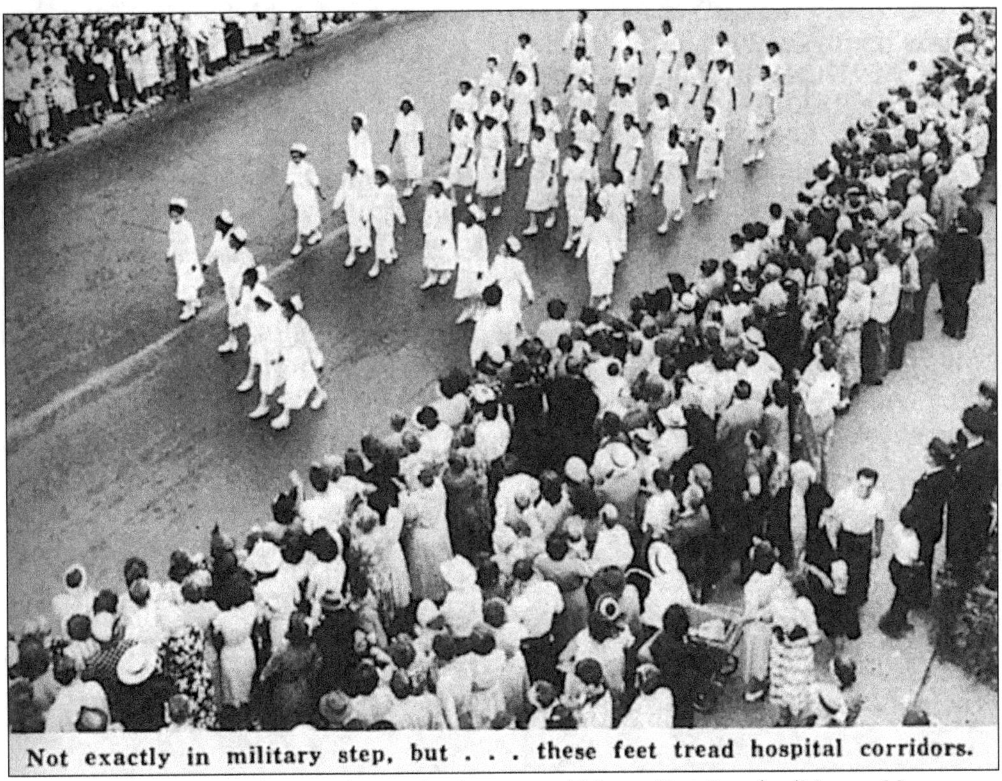

Not exactly in military step, but . . . these feet tread hospital corridors.

This is the procession of nurses during the first annual Nurses Day Parade. (*Novena Notes*, August 5, 1949, 11.)

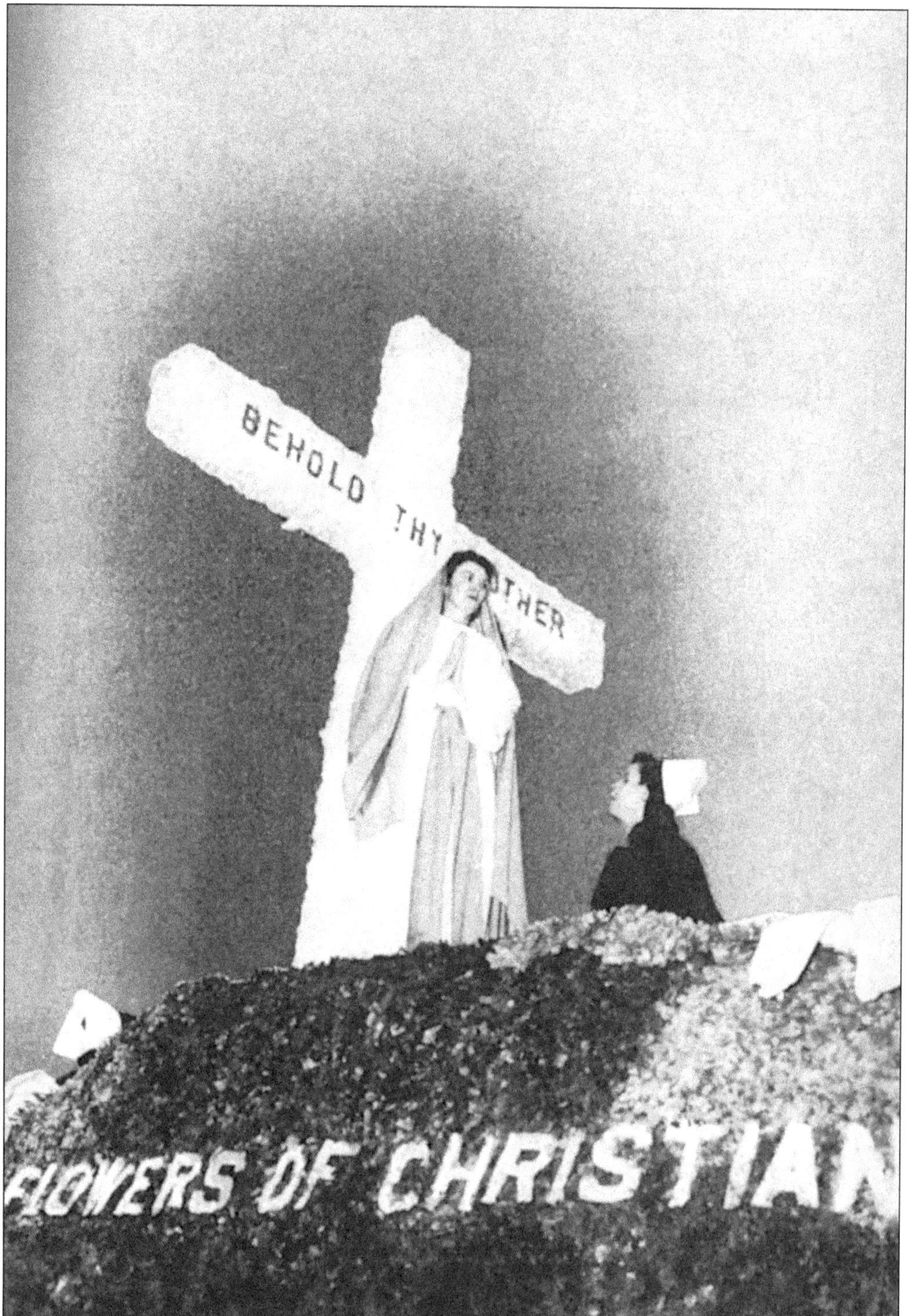

This *Novena Notes* cover of June 13, 1952, shows a close-up of the Novena float titled "First Nurse in Christendom." The cross on the top of the float was 17.5 feet tall.

Everyone agreed that the Nurses Day Parade in 1950 was a huge success and very effective in increasing the visibility of nurses. (*Novena Notes*, Oct. 6, 1950, 5.)

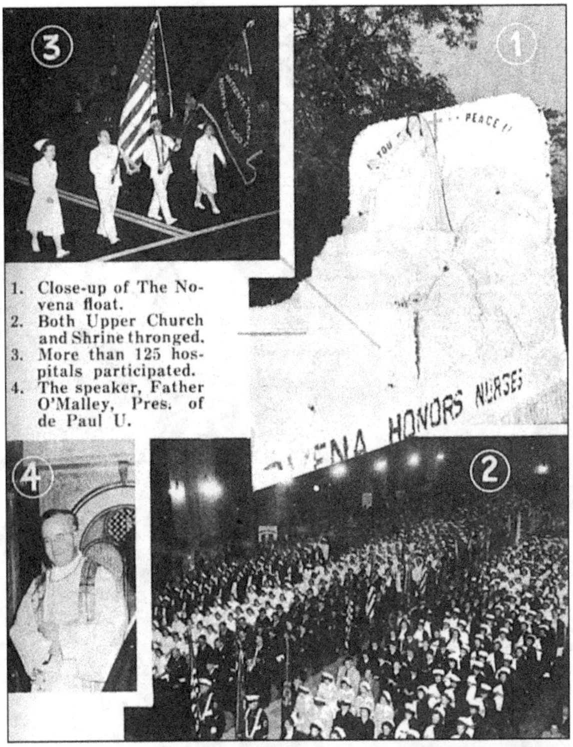

1. Close-up of The Novena float.
2. Both Upper Church and Shrine thronged.
3. More than 125 hospitals participated.
4. The speaker, Father O'Malley, Pres. of de Paul U.
HONORS NURSES

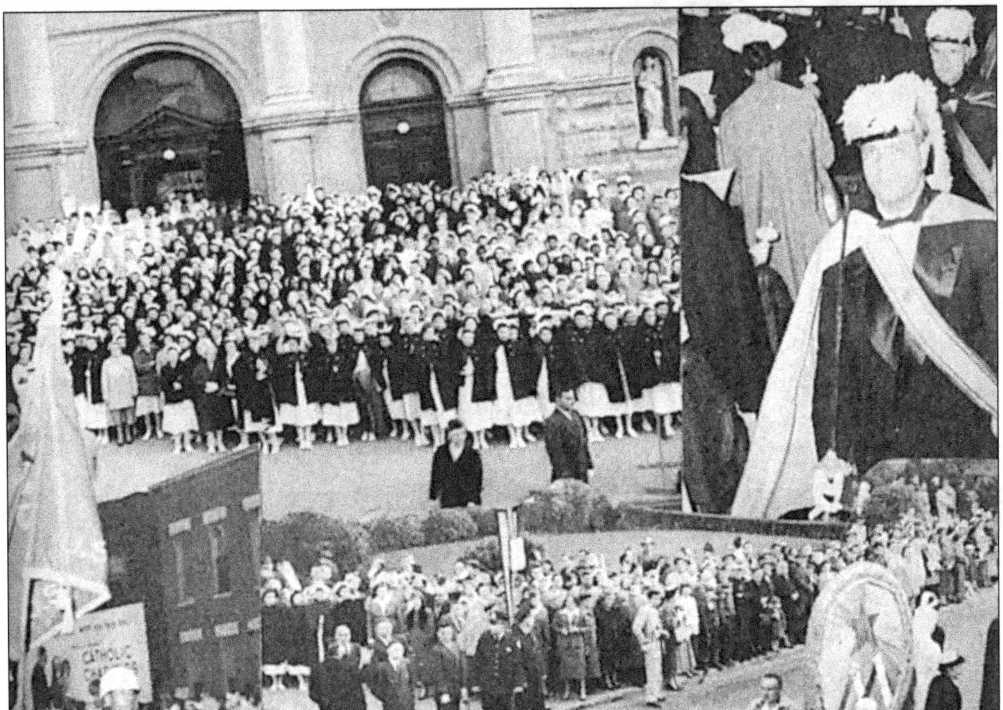

After each nursing unit finished marching, they gathered at the Novena Basilica to watch the balance of the parade. (*Novena Notes*, May 30, 1958, 5.)

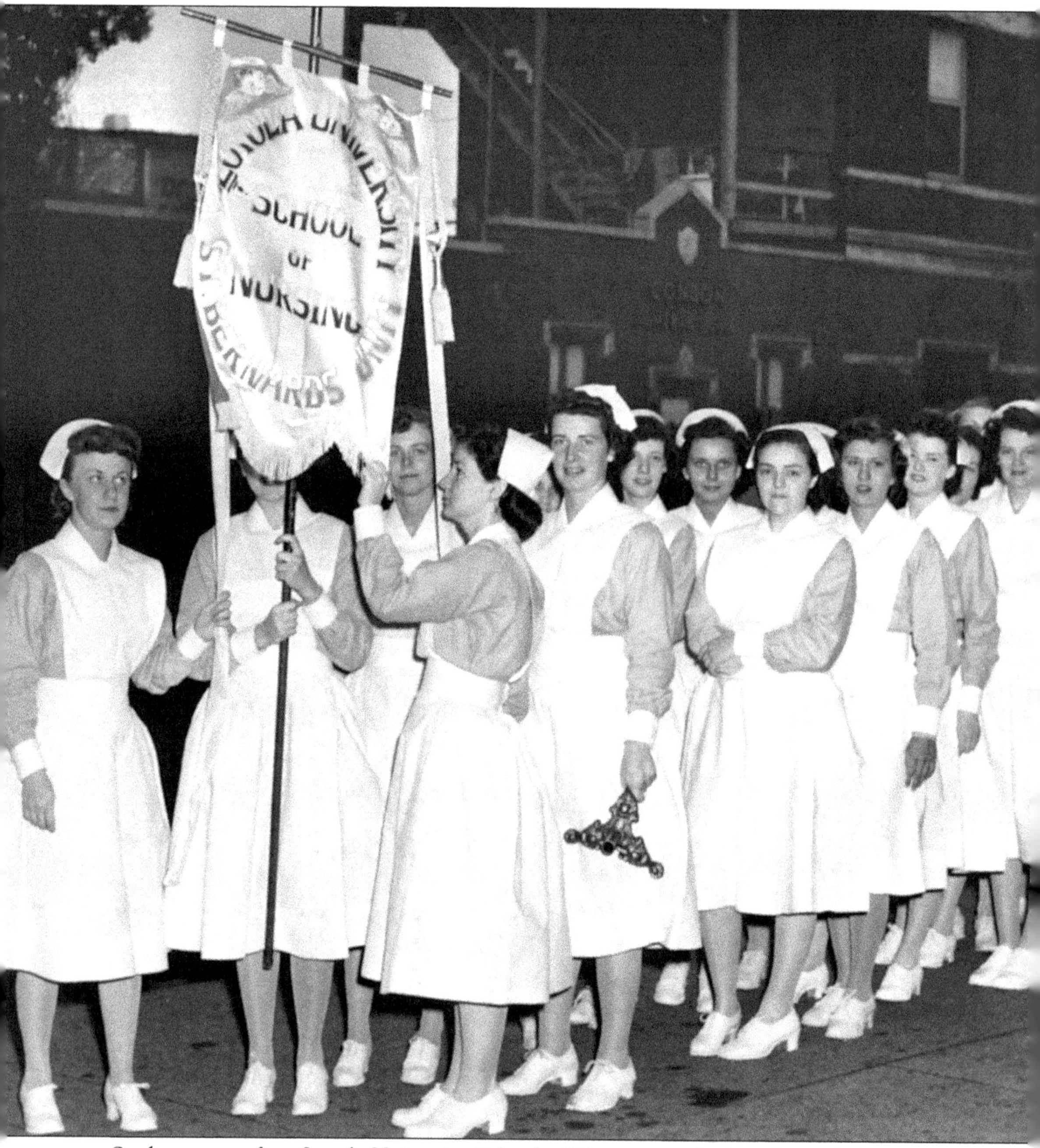

Student nurses from Loyola University School of Nursing marched in the prelude to the first Nurses Day Parade in 1948. (Photo also appeared in the *Novena Notes*, August 6, 1948, 8–9.)

Four

"If Only We Had a Nurse"

Parade Excitement

Each year between 1949–1958, the scene repeated itself. Spectators waited for the parade to begin with excitement and anticipation. The were anxious to see the first float go by, to hear the sounds of the first drumbeat and trumpet blast from the approaching marching band, and for the sight of over 2,000 "uniformed" nurses marching. Sometimes the nurses were in blue capes, sometimes in white uniforms and caps while others were in public health nursing uniforms or the nursing military dress of the service they represented. In every parade there were numerous student nurses marching in their schools' uniforms and caps. Church members, city and state government officials, merchants, media personalities, and communities united to visibly honor the unsung heroes of nursing.

From the beginning in 1949, every parade had prancing horses, floats, ambulances, and every type of mobile hospital imaginable—soldiers, sailors, marines, legionnaires, priests, nurses, and nursing students—all participating to show respect to nurses who care and provide service to those in need. More than 50 hospitals were represented at the first Nurses Day Parade. Heralded as "the World's Largest, Shortest Parade," the parade immortalized the contributions of countless men and women who provided competent, compassionate, quality healthcare to those in need. The parade was a public way to honor and demonstrate respect for a silent and somewhat invisible profession—nursing.

In 1949, society was suffering a severe nursing shortage that did not dissipate and would be repeated in the future. The shortage of nurses prompted Father Brissette to initiate the parade. In an announcement of the 1957 ninth annual Nurses Day Parade, it was stated that a minimum of 600,000 nurses were needed by 1970. It was anticipated that 300 nurses were required for every 100,000 individuals. It was hoped that by having a parade highlighting nurses and the extremely valuable service they provide, others would be inspired to become nurses and nurses would feel respected and honored.

It was hoped that in lonely hours watching by bedsides, or in trying moments calling for the utmost patience, memories of the sight and sound of the parade would help nurses to realize how much the public appreciated their vocation. (*Novena Notes*, June 11, 1954.)

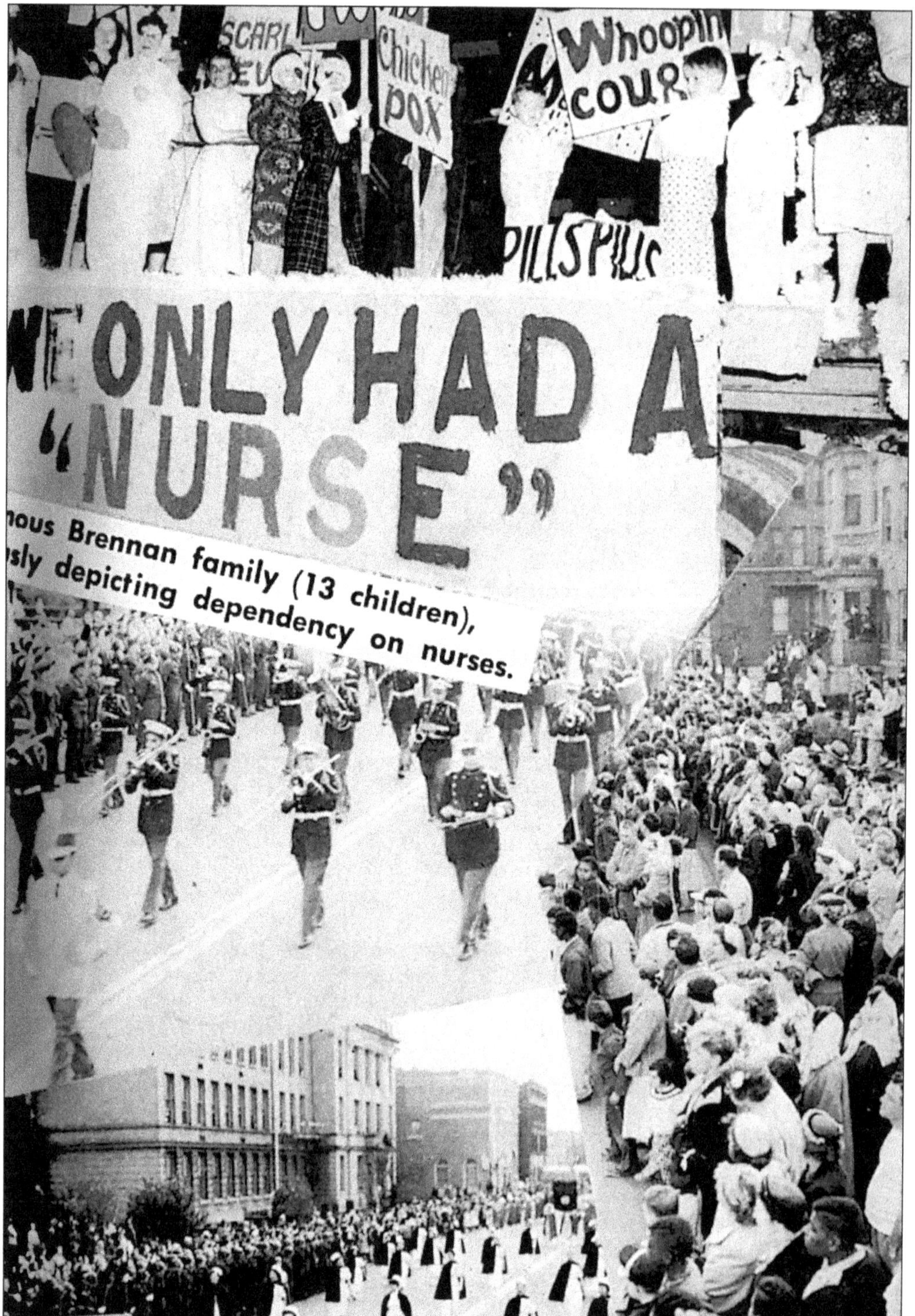
Chicken pox
Whoopin coug
PILLSPILLS
ONLY HAD A "NURSE"
ous Brennan family (13 children),
sly depicting dependency on nurses.

The Brennan family, who had 13 children, created a float demonstrating the importance of nurses to their families as well as to other families. The oldest Brennan girl became a nurse. (*Novena Sides*, *Novena Notes*, May 18, 1956, 12.) (Photo from *Novena Notes*, June 8, 1956, 7.)

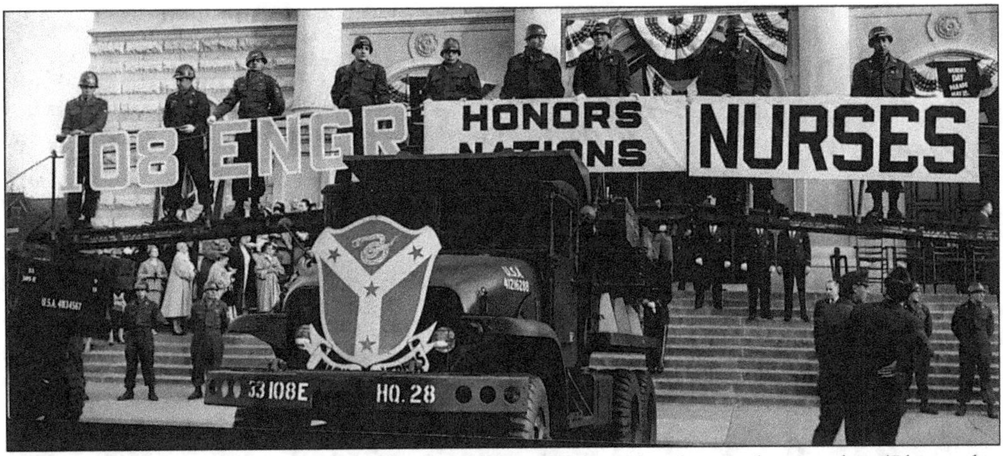

Nurses were honored by many different members of the public during the parades. (Photo also appeared in *Novena Notes*, June 8, 1956, cover.)

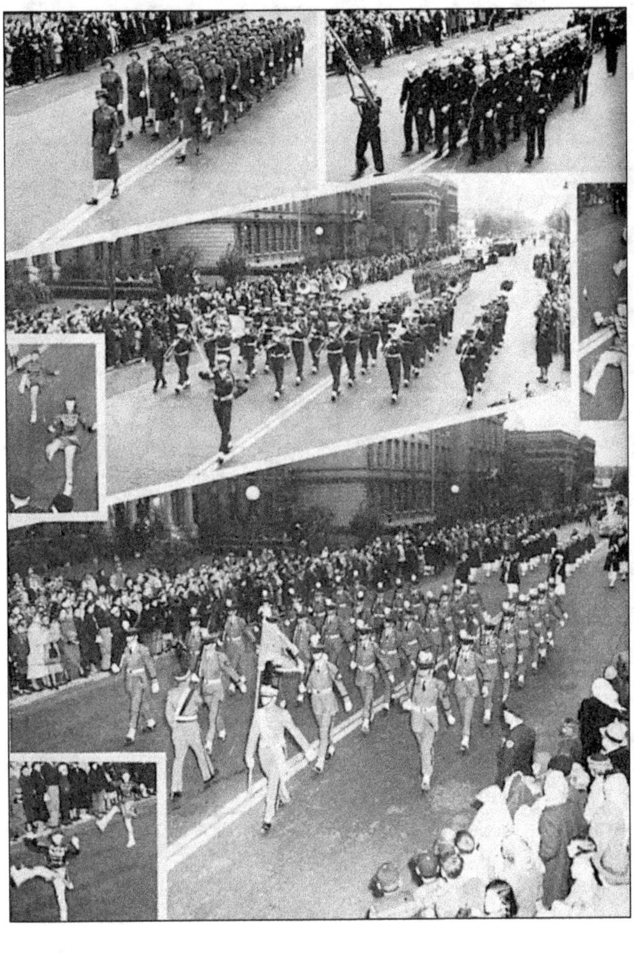

After the 1953 parade, the Coca-Cola Company provided 5,000 free Cokes to the marchers. (*Novena Notes*, June 12, 1953, 4.)

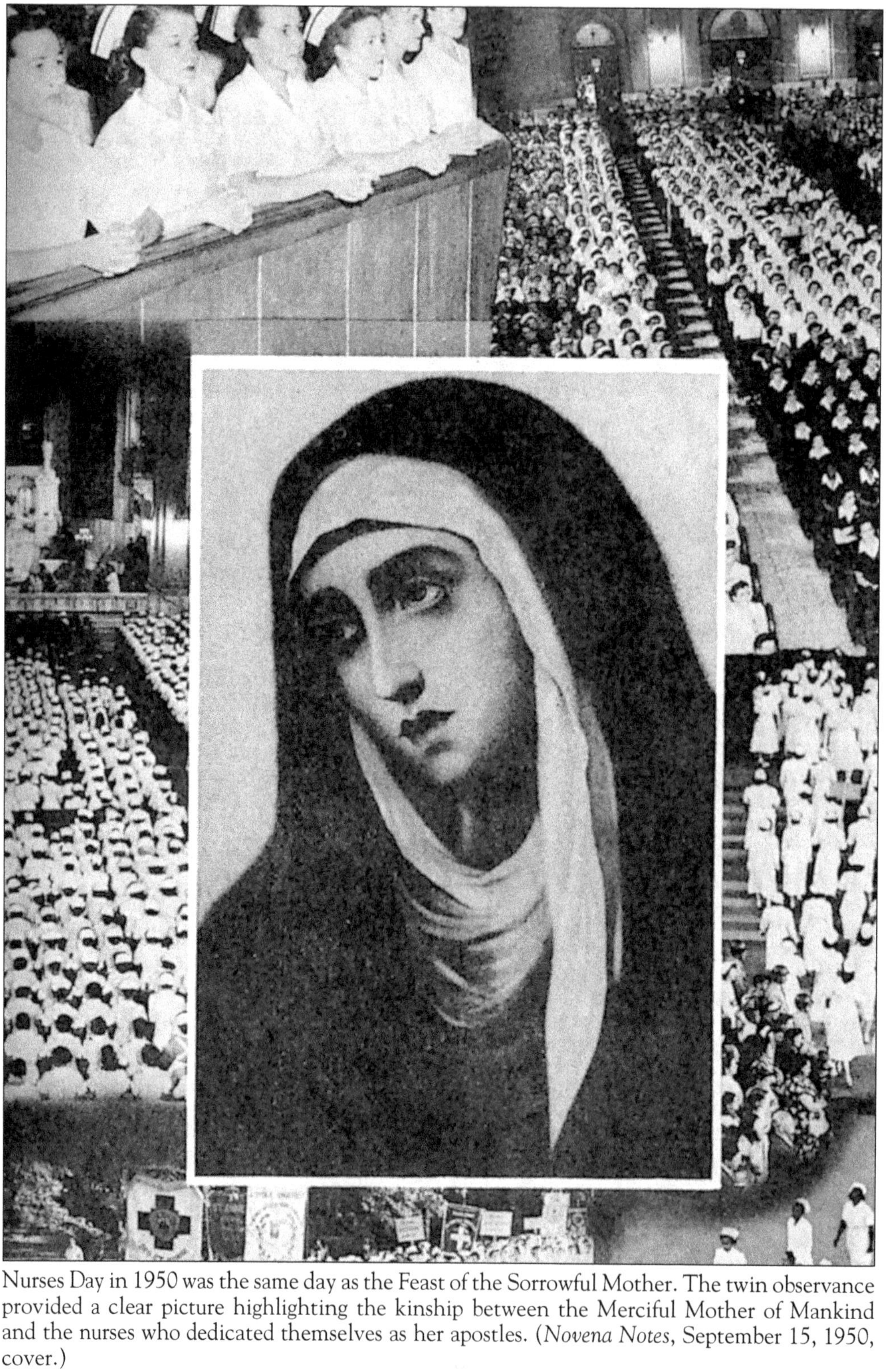

Nurses Day in 1950 was the same day as the Feast of the Sorrowful Mother. The twin observance provided a clear picture highlighting the kinship between the Merciful Mother of Mankind and the nurses who dedicated themselves as her apostles. (*Novena Notes*, September 15, 1950, cover.)

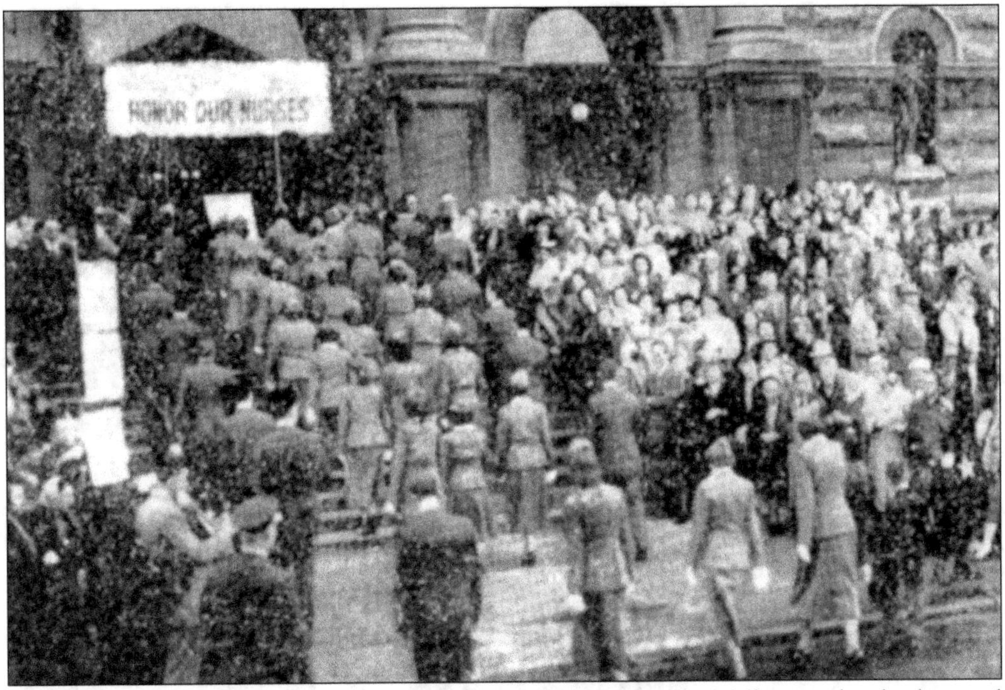
HONOR OUR NURSES
Pictured in May of 1951, nurses enter Our Lady of Sorrows Basilica following the third annual Chicago Nurses Day Parade.

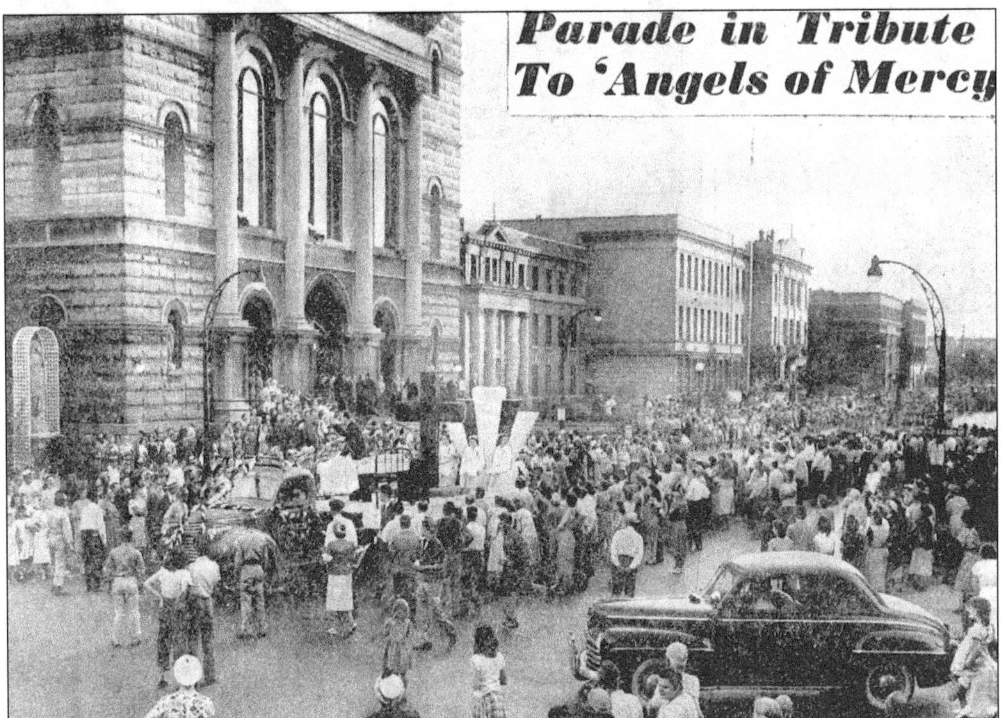
Parade in Tribute
To 'Angels of Mercy
Crowds jam the street outside of the National Shrine following the July 15, 1949 Nurses Day Parade. (*Chicago Daily News*, July 16, 1949)

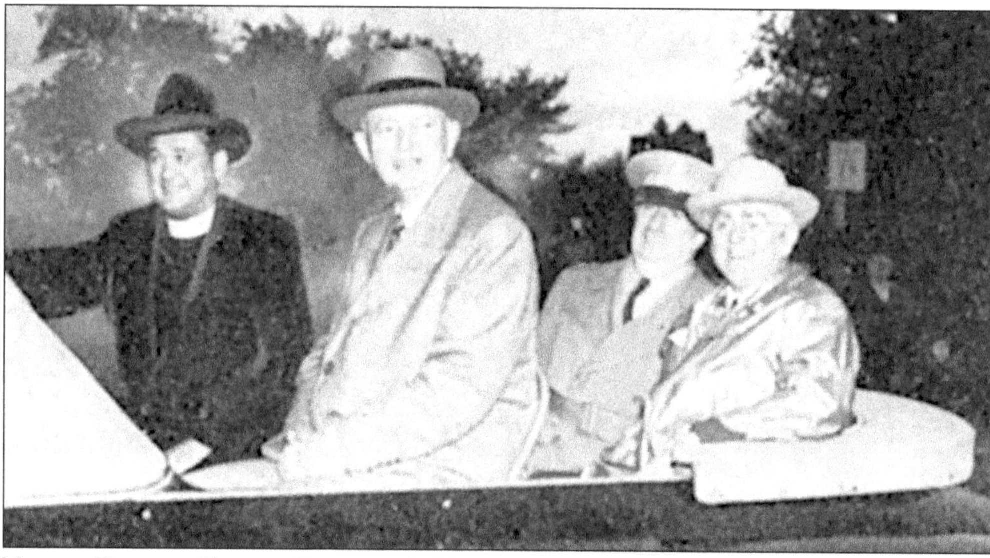

Novena Director Clarence Brissette, O.S.M., Mayor Kennelly, Major General Ferry (Grand Marshall), and Dr. Bundeson, head of the Chicago Health Department, are shown in the 1953 parade. (*Novena Notes*, June 12, 1953, 3.)

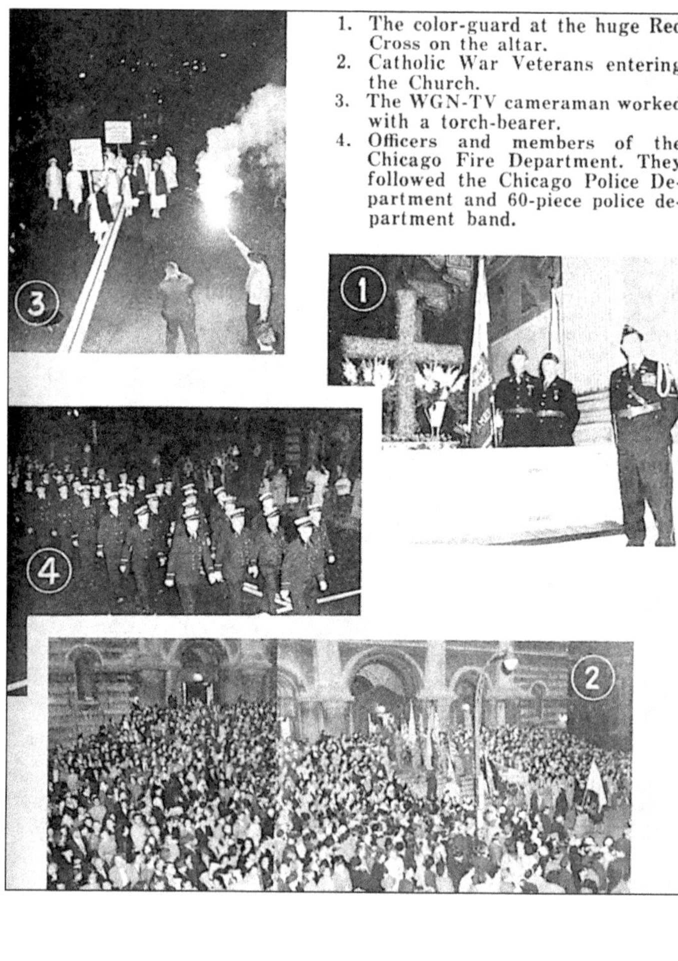

1. The color-guard at the huge Red Cross on the altar.
2. Catholic War Veterans entering the Church.
3. The WGN-TV cameraman worked with a torch-bearer.
4. Officers and members of the Chicago Fire Department. They followed the Chicago Police Department and 60-piece police department band.

The Chicago police provided a 60-person marching band to perform for the 1950 parade. (*Novena Notes*, October 6, 1950, 11.)

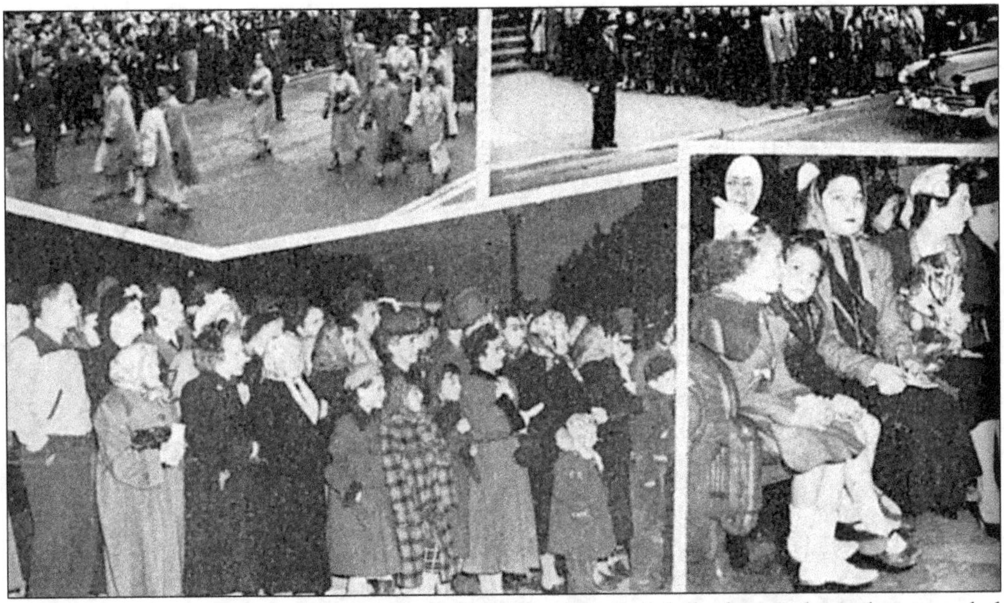

Chicagoans "love a parade." Chicago's 1953 Nurses Day Parade had everything that appealed to parade-goers. Leading the parade was the 33rd Division Band, Infantry, Medical Corps, army nurses, WACs, marines, Great Lakes Naval Band, sailors, navy nurses, and WAVES, along with the Red Cross, Chicago police band, and firemen. Crowds line up six and seven people deep along the parade route. (*Novena Notes*, June 12, 1953, 2.)

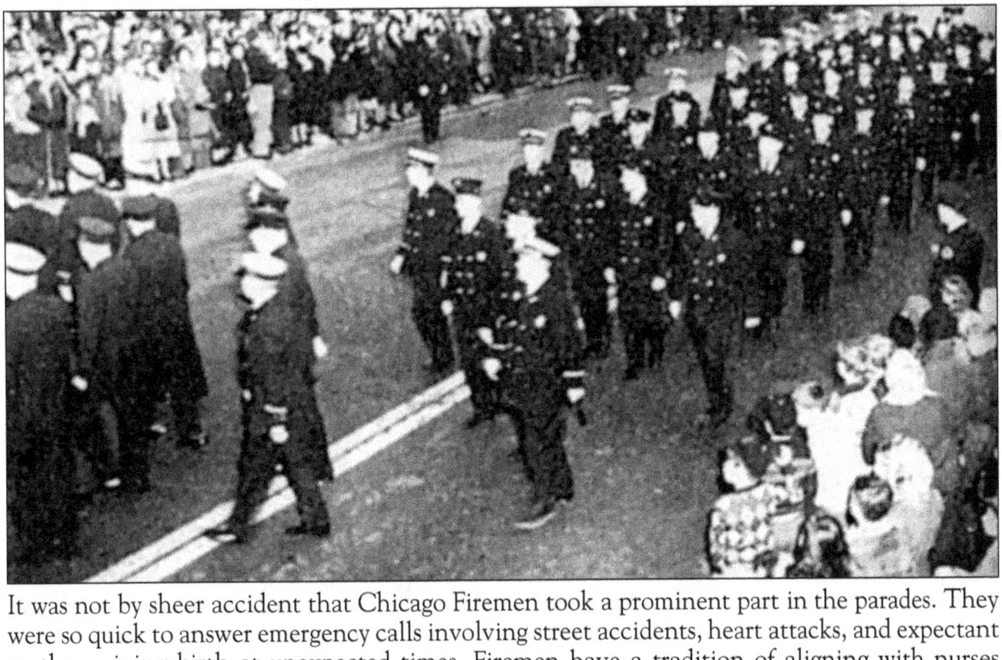

It was not by sheer accident that Chicago Firemen took a prominent part in the parades. They were so quick to answer emergency calls involving street accidents, heart attacks, and expectant mothers giving birth at unexpected times. Firemen have a tradition of aligning with nurses during emergencies. The firemen knew the difficulties of getting private nurses in time of emergency and they wanted to honor the "angels of mercy." (*Novena Notes*, June 12, 1953, 2.)

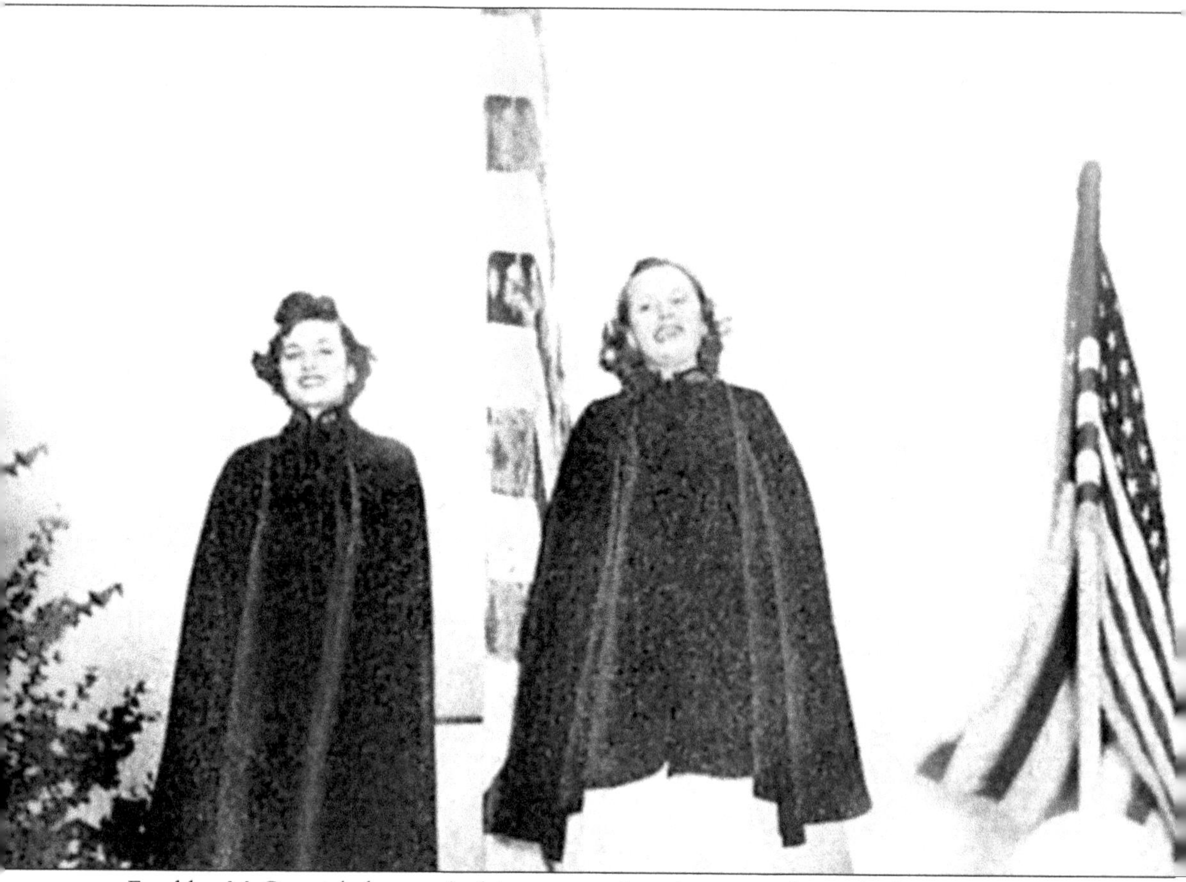

Franklyn McCormick, known for his poetry and readings on radio and television, narrated the significance of parade scenes for WCFL studios. After the Chicago-Detroit night baseball game was over on May 22, 1953, the parade narrations were broadcast nationwide. Nurses were proud of both their profession and of their country, as the parade provides a platform for national visability. (*Novena Notes*, June 12, 1953, 11.)

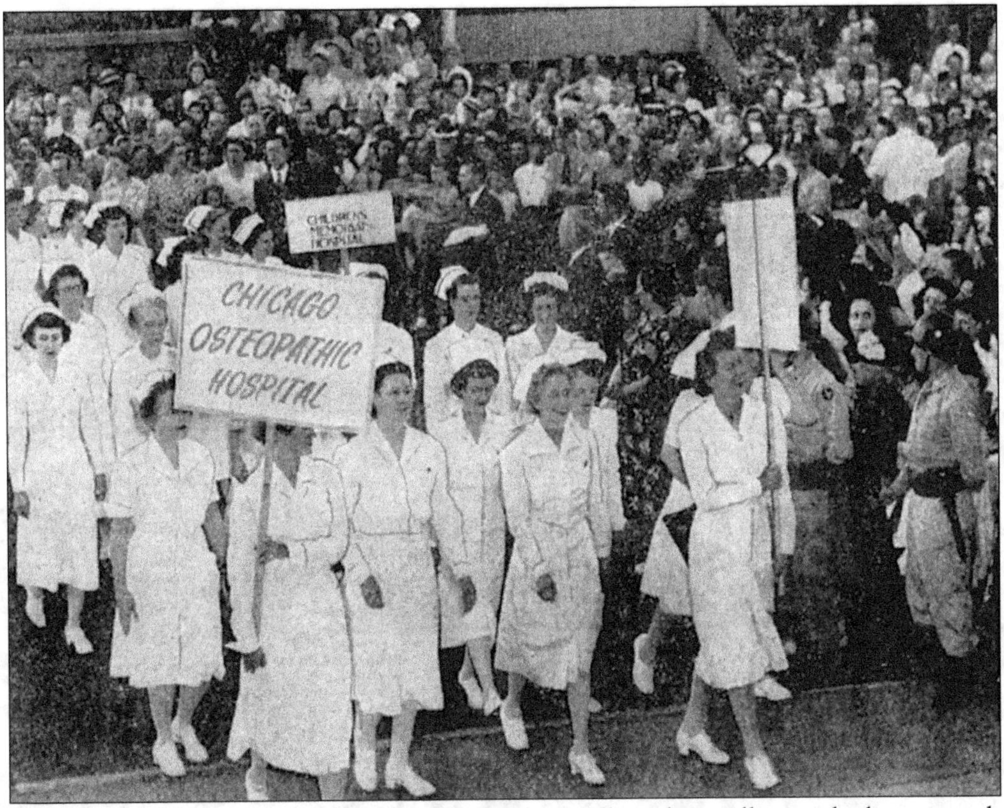

Nurses from Chicago Osteopathic Hospital march proudly and stoically pass the honor guards while entering Our Lady of Sorrows Basilica. (*Chicago Daily News*, July 16, 1949)

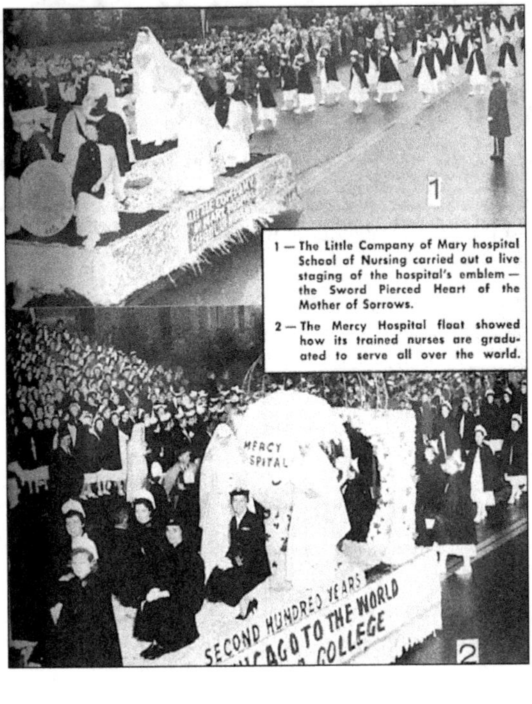

The rain was so heavy prior to the parade beginning on May 10, 1957, that a bus load of nurses arrived from St. Francis Hospital in Milwaukee, Wisconsin, at three in the afternoon and camped in their bus until the parade began at seven in the evening. When the parade began, the rain stopped, and floats and marchers started appearing. (John Long, *Novena Notes*, May 31, 1957, 6.)

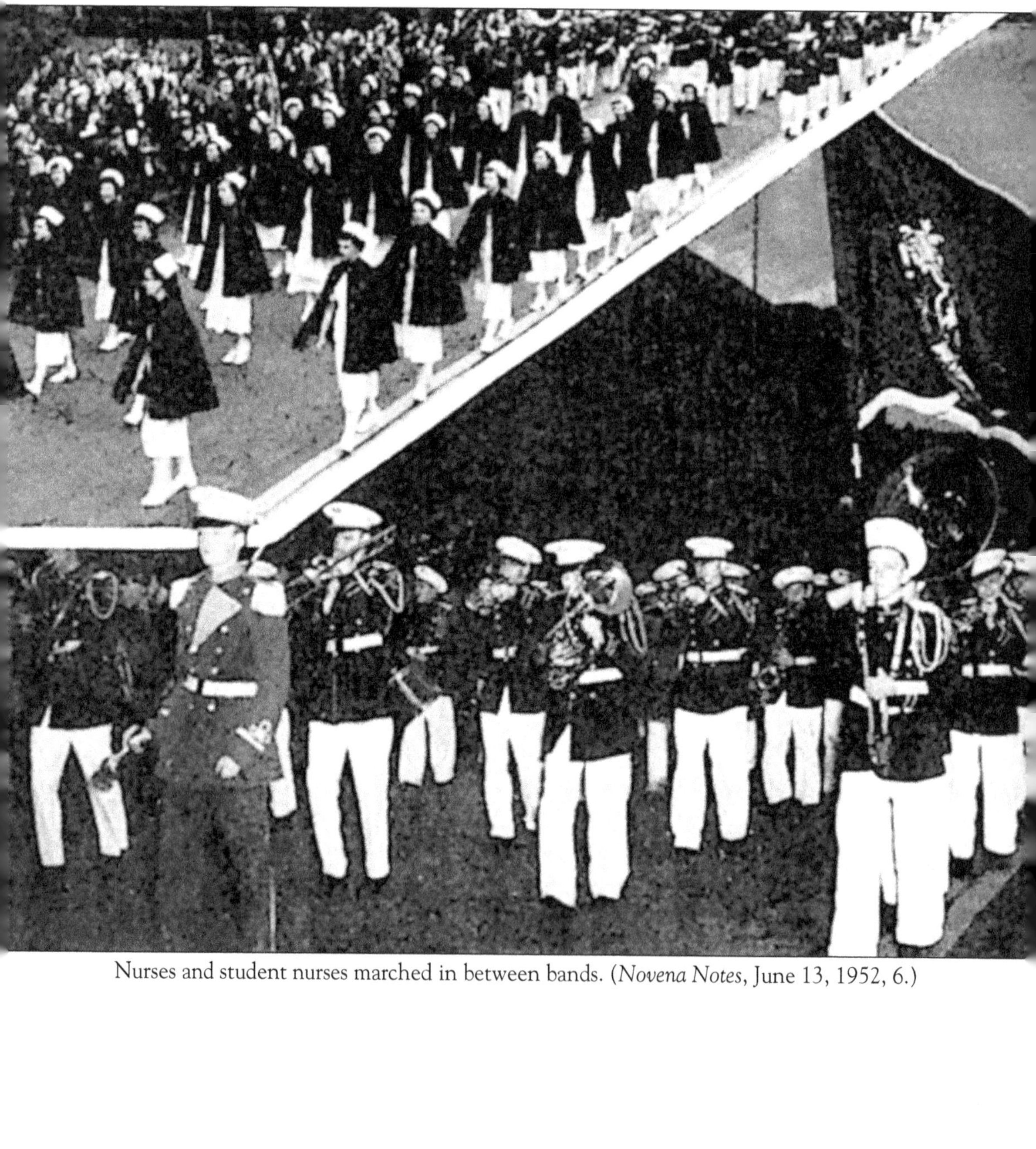

Nurses and student nurses marched in between bands. (*Novena Notes*, June 13, 1952, 6.)

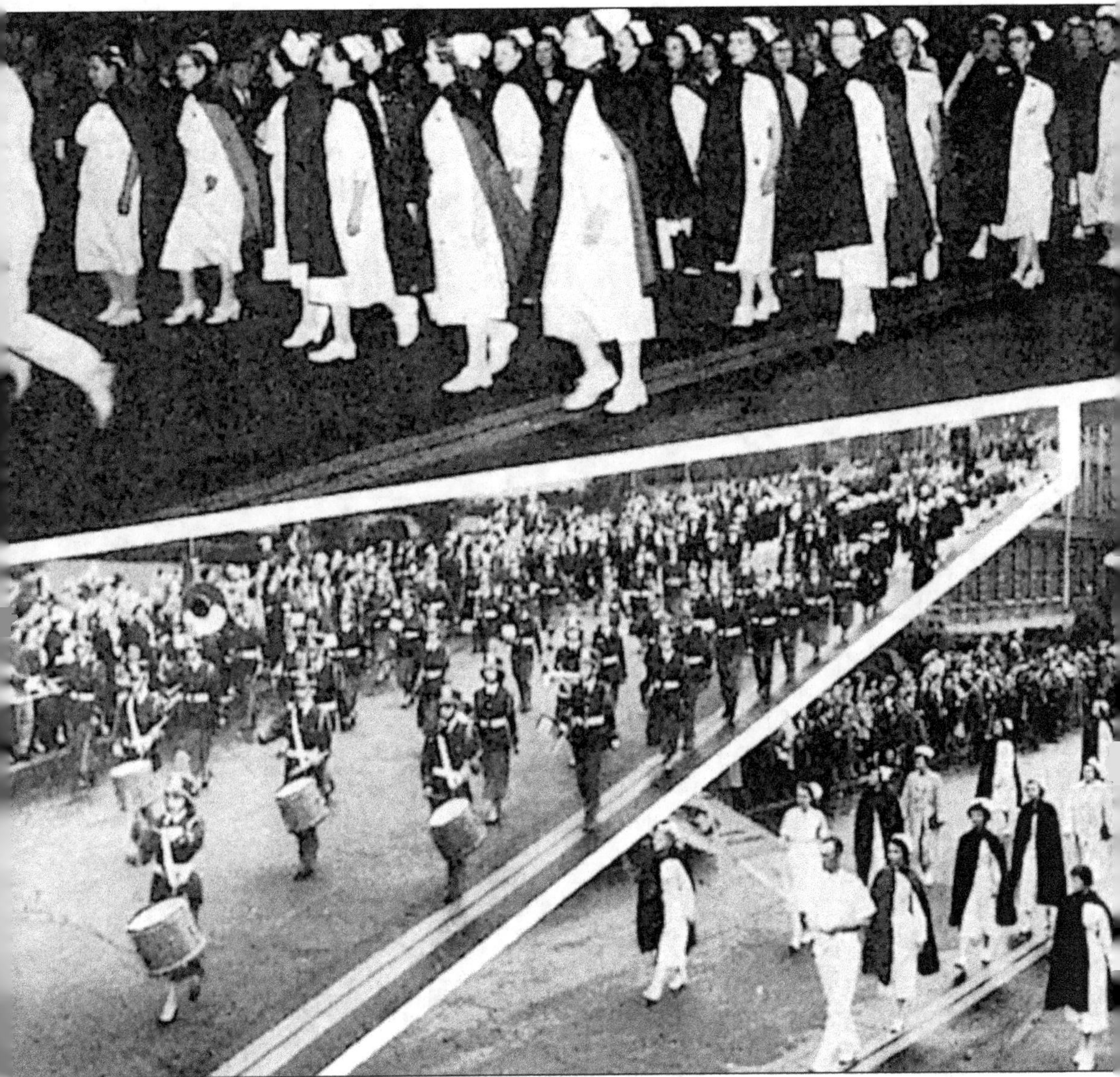

The rhythm of marching bands from government services and local high schools was interspersed with the marching nurses. (*Novena Notes*, June 13, 1952, 6.)

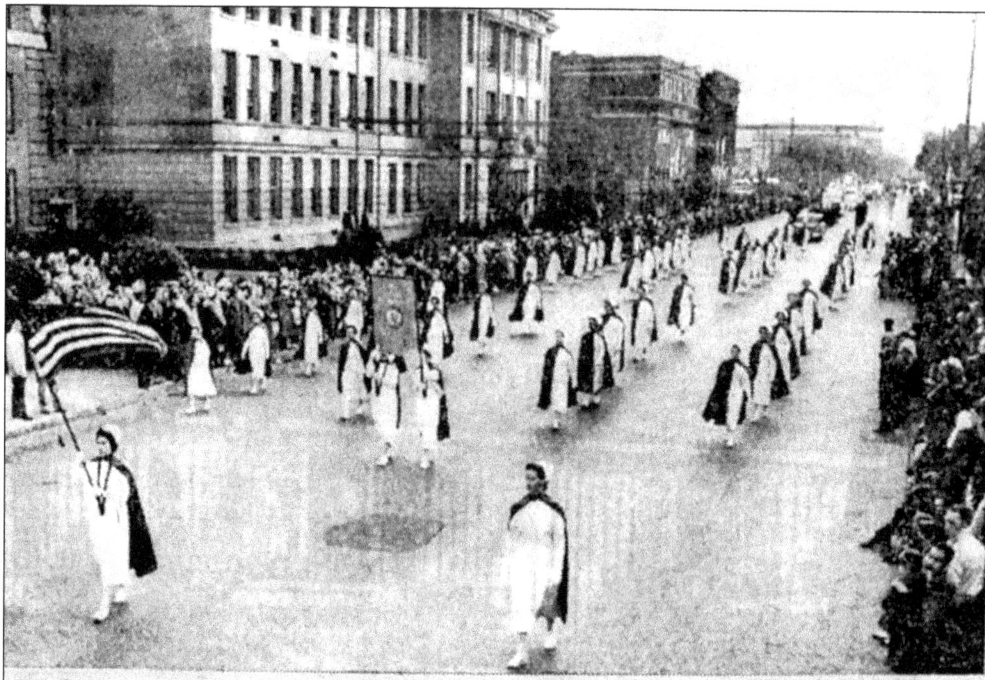

[TRIBUNE Photo]

Part of the 2,000 nurses marching in Jackson boulevard yesterday as part of ceremonies of enth annual Nurses' day. More than 2,000 other marchers participated in the event.

40,000 Turn Out for Annual Marching

Two thousand uniformed nurses, their capes fluttering in the chill evening air, marched down Jackson boulevard from Garfield park last night in a colorful hour-long parade.

The nurses were joined by 2,000 other marchers who included units, drill teams, massed colors, and bands from the army, navy, marines, national guard, and Chicago police and fire departments.

10th Annual Fete

It was the 10th annual Nurses day parade sponsored by the Sorrowful Mother novena of Our Lady of Sorrows basilica. The parade moved from Hamlin avenue and Jackson boulevard east to the basilica, 3121 Jackson blvd., as an estimated 40,000 spectators lined the street.

A group of dignitaries viewed the marchers from the steps of the basilica. They included the Rev. Alphonse Monta, superior general of the Servite order of priests from Rome; Dr. Herman Bundesen president of the Chicago board of health; and Dr. Otto Bettag, state welfare director

It is Non-Denominational

It was a non-denominational parade which paid tribute to nurses representing hospitals from thruout the Chicago area and those as far distant as Milwaukee.

The annual parade, said to be the only one of its kind in the world, was conceived a decade ago to call attention to a shortage of nurses in all categories and to emphasize the high dedication plane in the nursing field.

The marchers were led by the 5th army band, followed by a float honoring Florence Nightingale, founder of modern nursing.

Flags on Posts

American flags were draped on lamp posts along the line of march.

As the parade broke up, nurses of the Roman Catholic faith entered the basilica for novena services. The Rev. James Moscow, assistant director of Catholic hospitals in the Chicago archdiocese, spoke at the services.

Over 40,000 spectators turned out to honor 2,000 nurses marching in the "Twilight Spectacular." (*Chicago Daily Tribune*, May 10, 1958.)

Here, the *Chicago Daily Sun-Times* reports on the upcoming 1956 parade.

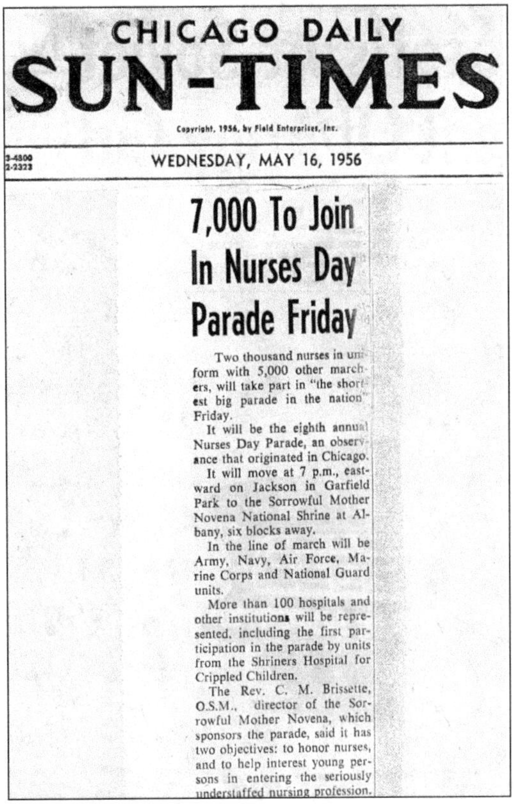

CHICAGO DAILY

SUN-TIMES

Copyright, 1956, by Field Enterprises, Inc.

3-4800 2-2323 WEDNESDAY, MAY 16, 1956

7,000 To Join In Nurses Day Parade Friday

Two thousand nurses in uniform with 5,000 other marchers, will take part in "the shortest big parade in the nation" Friday.

It will be the eighth annual Nurses Day Parade, an observance that originated in Chicago.

It will move at 7 p.m., eastward on Jackson in Garfield Park to the Sorrowful Mother Novena National Shrine at Albany, six blocks away.

In the line of march will be Army, Navy, Air Force, Marine Corps and National Guard units.

More than 100 hospitals and other institutions will be represented, including the first participation in the parade by units from the Shriners Hospital for Crippled Children.

The Rev. C. M. Brissette, O.S.M., director of the Sorrowful Mother Novena, which sponsors the parade, said it has two objectives: to honor nurses, and to help interest young persons in entering the seriously understaffed nursing profession.

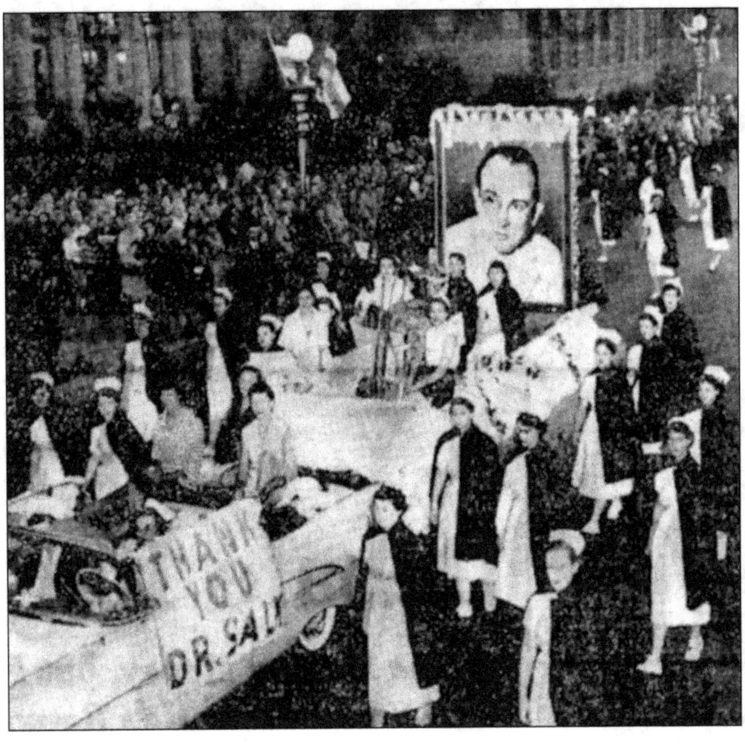

St. Elizabeth Hospital's School of Nursing float honored Dr. Jonas Salk. (*Chicago Daily News*, May 21, 1955)

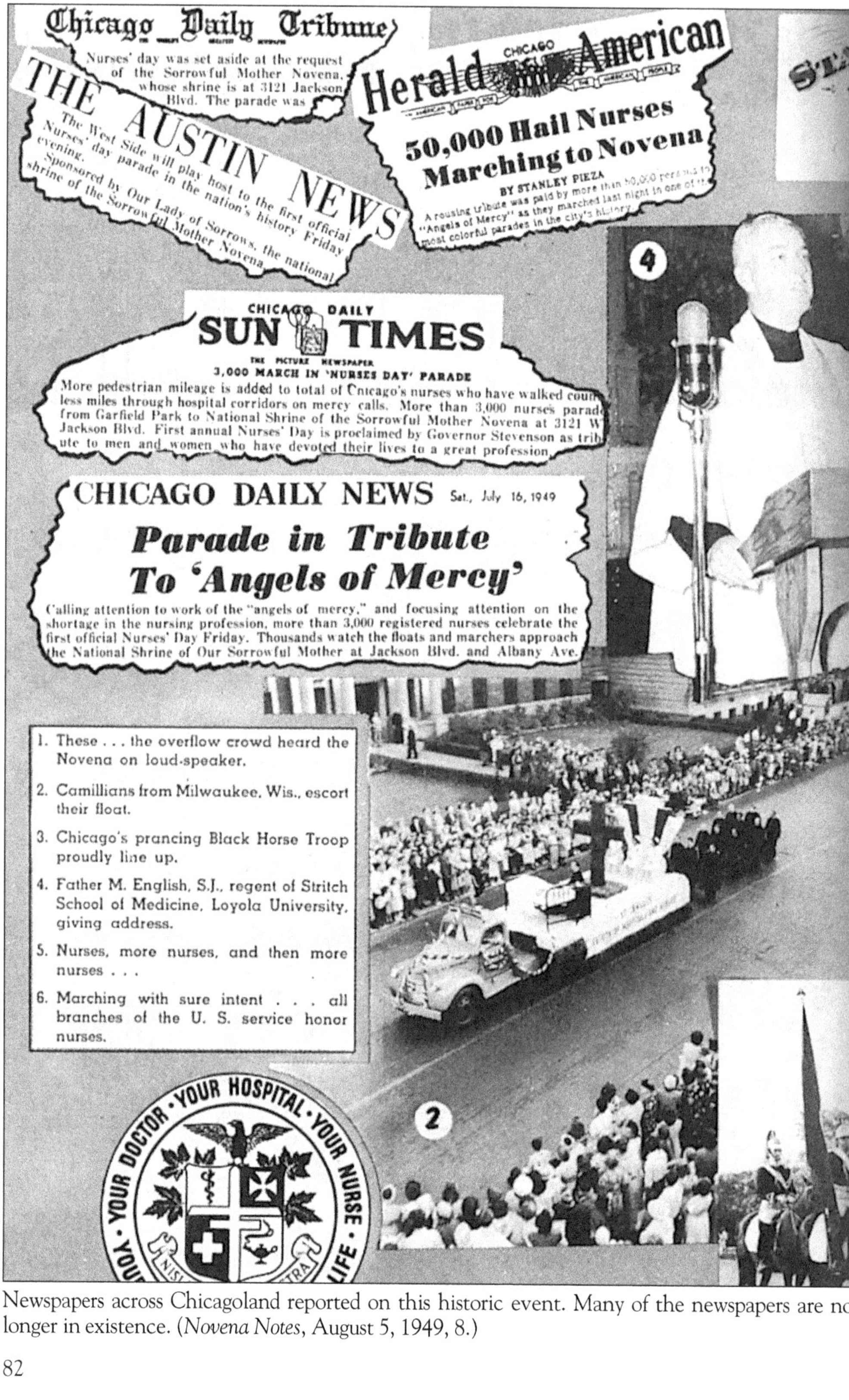

Chicago Daily Tribune

Nurses' day was set aside at the request of the Sorrowful Mother Novena, whose shrine is at 3121 Jackson Blvd. The parade was

THE AUSTIN NEWS

The West Side will play host to the first official Nurses' day parade in the nation's history Friday evening.

Sponsored by Our Lady of Sorrows, the national shrine of the Sorrowful Mother Novena.

Chicago Herald-American

50,000 Hail Nurses Marching to Novena

BY STANLEY PIEZA

A rousing tribute was paid by more than 50,000 persons to "Angels of Mercy" as they marched last night in one of the most colorful parades in the city's history.

CHICAGO DAILY SUN-TIMES

THE PICTURE NEWSPAPER

3,000 MARCH IN 'NURSES DAY' PARADE

More pedestrian mileage is added to total of Chicago's nurses who have walked coun less miles through hospital corridors on mercy calls. More than 3,000 nurses parad from Garfield Park to National Shrine of the Sorrowful Mother Novena at 3121 W Jackson Blvd. First annual Nurses' Day is proclaimed by Governor Stevenson as trib ute to men and women who have devoted their lives to a great profession.

CHICAGO DAILY NEWS Sat., July 16, 1949

Parade in Tribute To 'Angels of Mercy'

Calling attention to work of the "angels of mercy," and focusing attention on the shortage in the nursing profession, more than 3,000 registered nurses celebrate the first official Nurses' Day Friday. Thousands watch the floats and marchers approach the National Shrine of Our Sorrowful Mother at Jackson Blvd. and Albany Ave.

1. These . . . the overflow crowd heard the Novena on loud-speaker.
2. Camillians from Milwaukee, Wis., escort their float.
3. Chicago's prancing Black Horse Troop proudly line up.
4. Father M. English, S.J., regent of Stritch School of Medicine, Loyola University, giving address.
5. Nurses, more nurses, and then more nurses . . .
6. Marching with sure intent . . . all branches of the U. S. service honor nurses.

Newspapers across Chicagoland reported on this historic event. Many of the newspapers are no longer in existence. (*Novena Notes*, August 5, 1949, 8.)

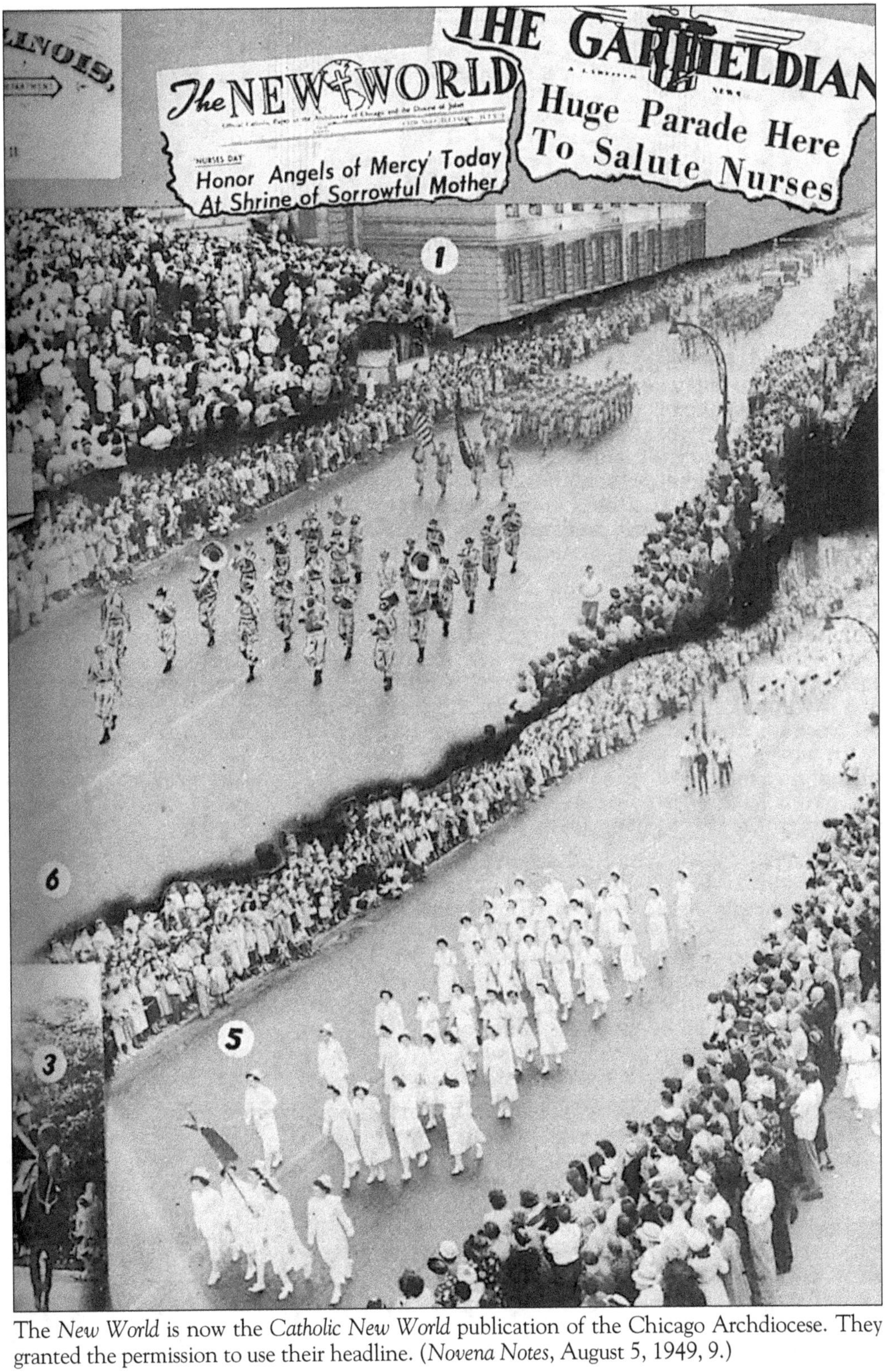
The NEW WORLD
NURSES DAY
Honor Angels of Mercy' Today
At Shrine of Sorrowful Mother
Huge Parade Here
To Salute Nurses
1
6
5
3

The *New World* is now the *Catholic New World* publication of the Chicago Archdiocese. They granted the permission to use their headline. (*Novena Notes*, August 5, 1949, 9.)

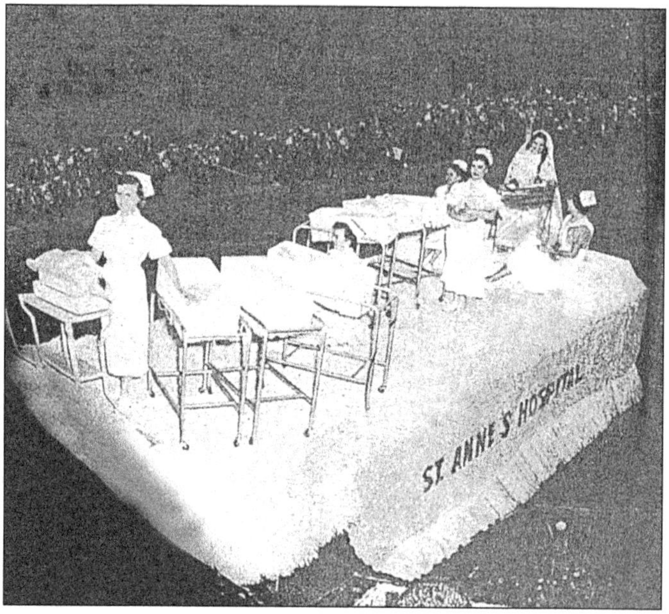

Floats were stories of how nurses cared for patients. (*Novena Notes*, June 10, 1955, 12.)

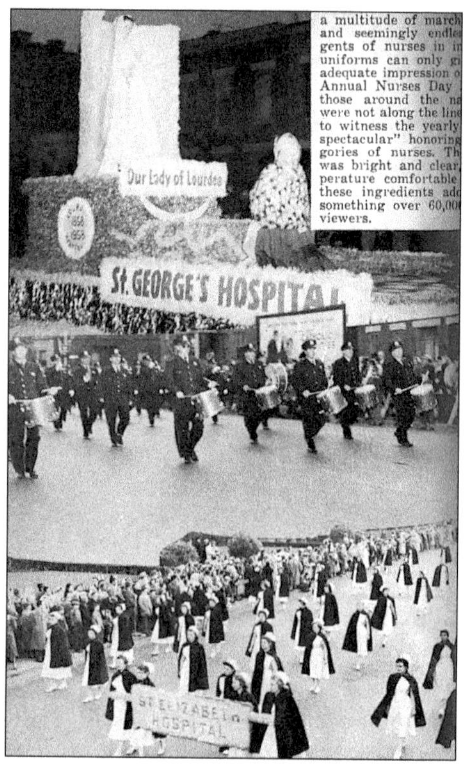
a multitude of march
and seemingly endl
gents of nurses in i
uniforms can only g
adequate impression o
Annual Nurses Day
those around the n
were not along the lin
to witness the yearly
spectacular" honorin
gories of nurses. Th
was bright and clear
perature comfortable
these ingredients ad
something over 60,00
viewers.
Our Lady of Lourdes
ST. GEORGE'S HOSPITAL

In 1958, the parade weather was bright with clear skies and comfortable temperatures, unlike the start of the parade in 1957, with cloudy skies after the rain. (*Novena Notes*, May 30, 1958, 4.)

The 1953 floats simulated nurses caring for patients and told a story of the nurses' work. (*Novena Notes*, June 12, 1953, 5.)

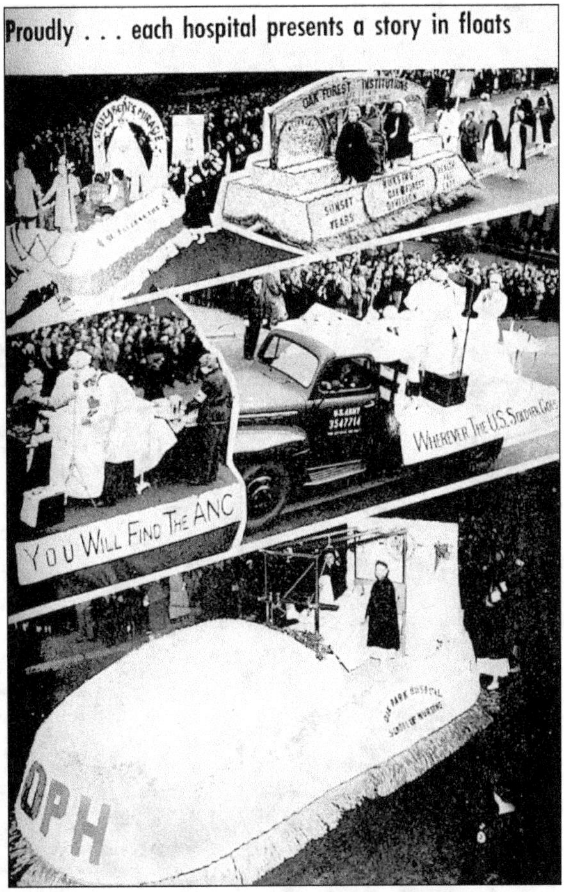
Proudly . . . each hospital presents a story in floats
OAK FOREST INSTITUTIONS
SUNSET YEARS
U.S. ARMY
WHEREVER THE U.S. SOLDIER
YOU WILL FIND THE ANC
OPH

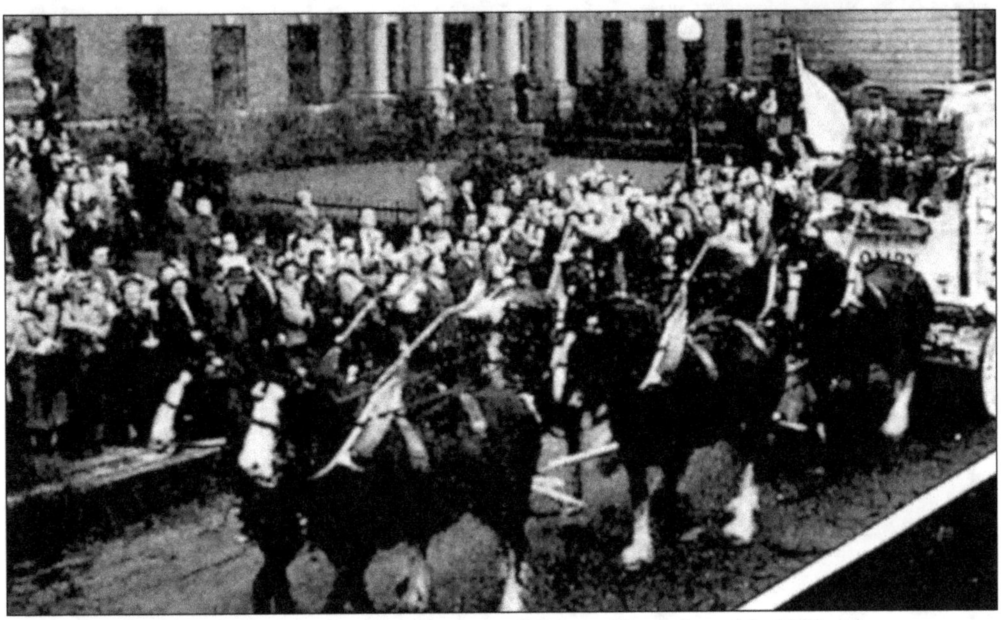

Prancing horses could be found in every parade. (*Novena Notes*, June 13, 1952, 4.)

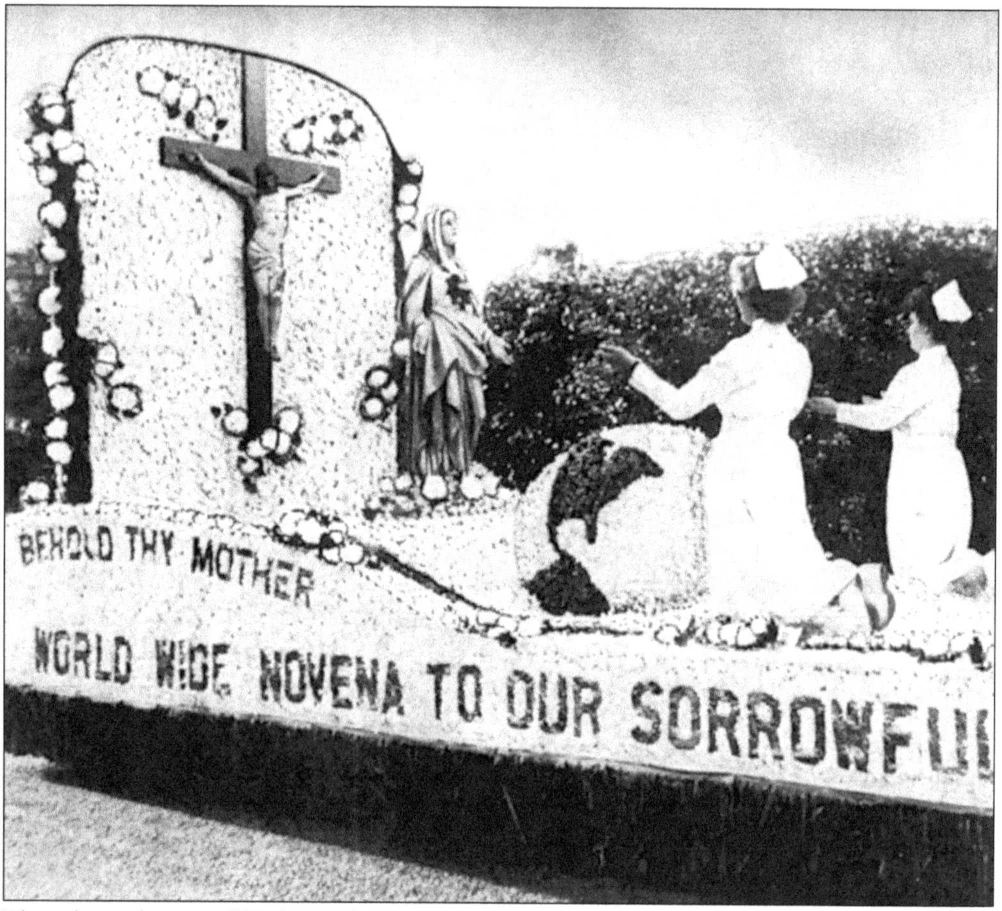

This photo shows a "World Wide Novena" float honoring Our Sorrowful Mother. (*Novena Notes*, August 5, 1949, cover.)

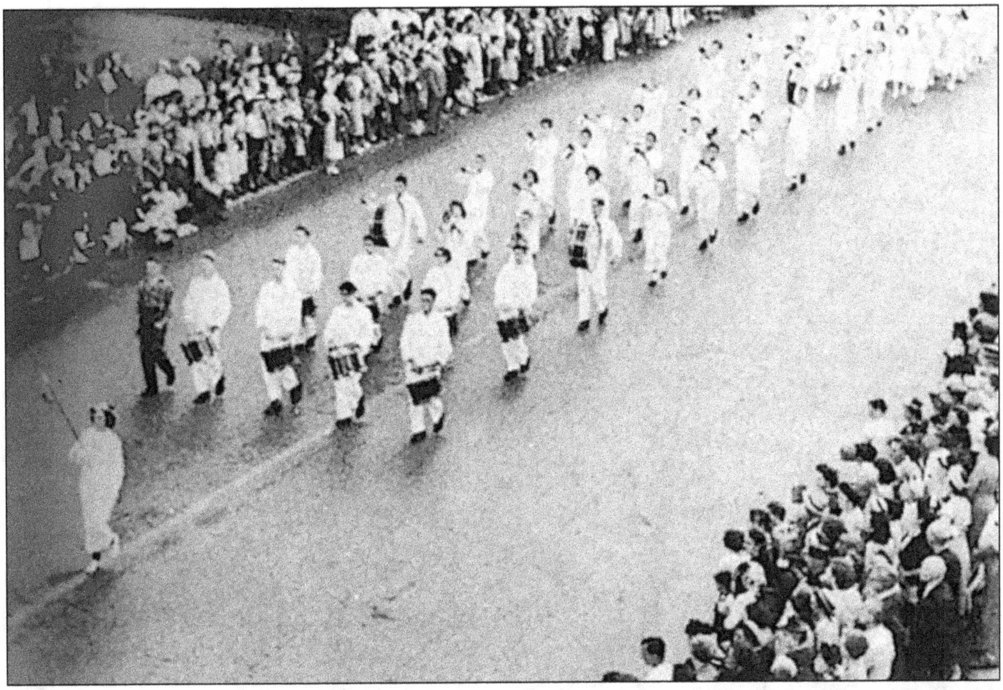

Crowds of 50,000 lined up three and four people deep to watch the colorful parade by the Novena National Shrine, July 1949. (*Novena Notes*, August 5, 1949, 7.)

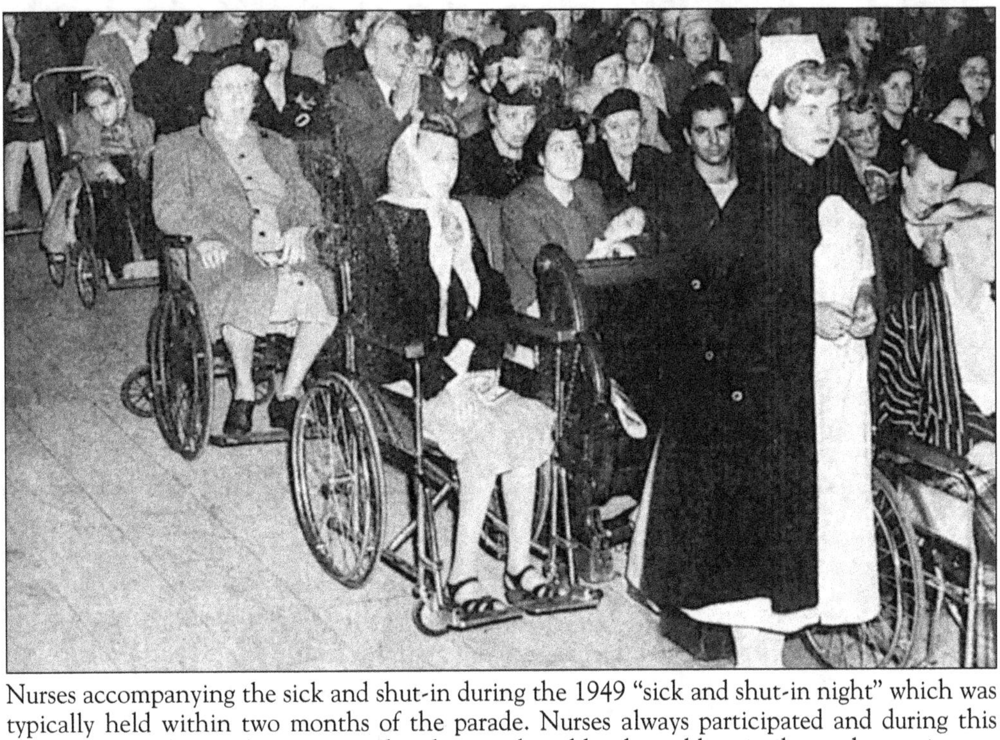

Nurses accompanying the sick and shut-in during the 1949 "sick and shut-in night" which was typically held within two months of the parade. Nurses always participated and during this night their work was also recognized and remembered by the public, similar to the sentiments displayed during the parade. (*Novena Notes*, Sept. 8, 1950, cover.)

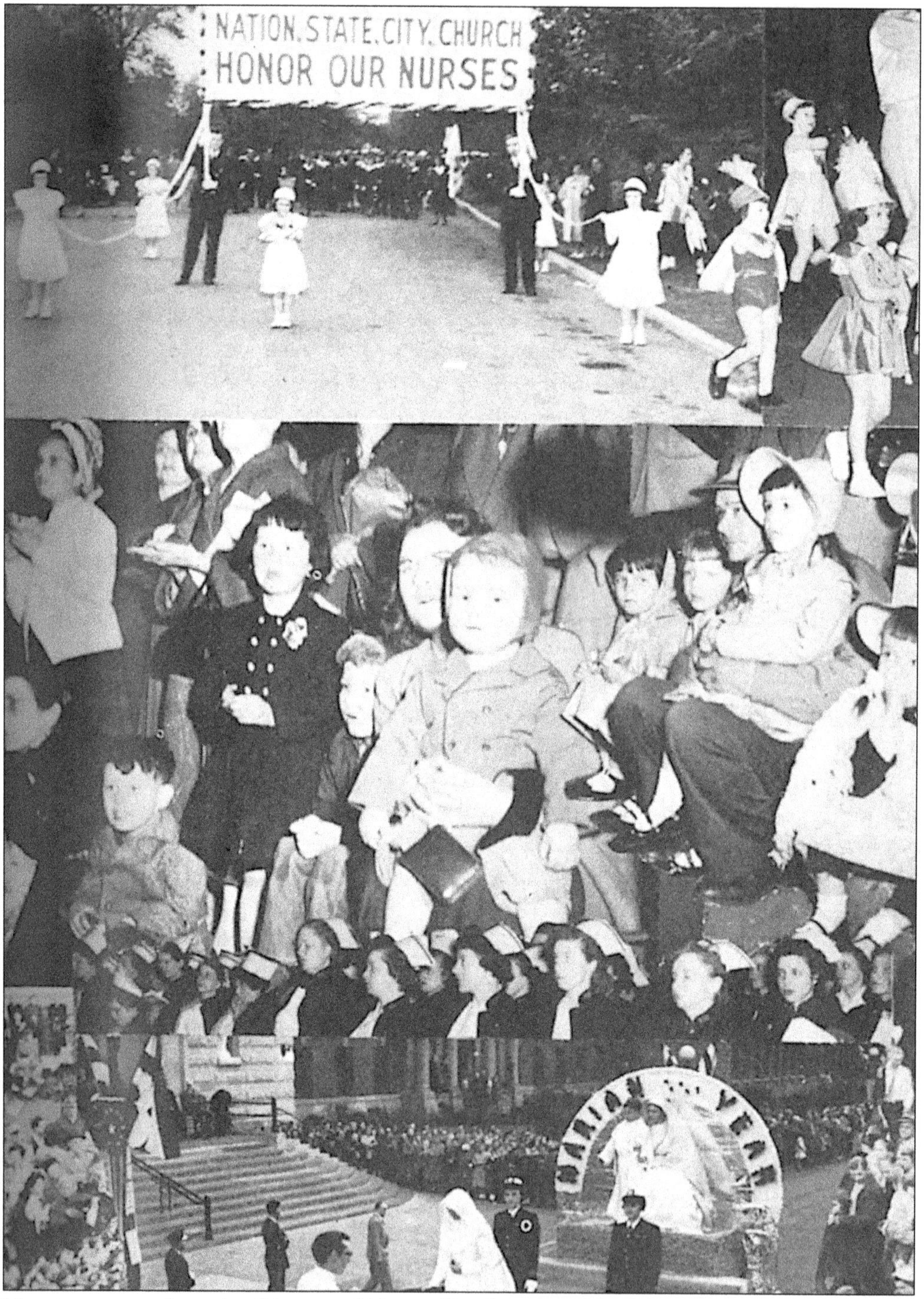

Here are scenes from the 6th annual Nurses Day Parade, 1954. More than 150 organizations were represented. The story-telling floats, prepared and entered by hospitals, brought continuous applause from the onlookers lining Jackson Boulevard. This was only the second time in 18 years that the whole issue of the *Novena Notes* was dedicated to pictures of the Nurses Day Parade. (*Novena Notes*, June 11, 1954, cover.)

Eighteen marching bands participated in the 1953 Nurses Day Parade. All of the Chicago Metropolitan newspapers covered the parade, along with WGN-TV. Mr. Landwehr, editor of the *Garfieldian*, gave the Nurses Day Parade front page headlines. (*Novena Notes*, June 12, 1953, 7.)

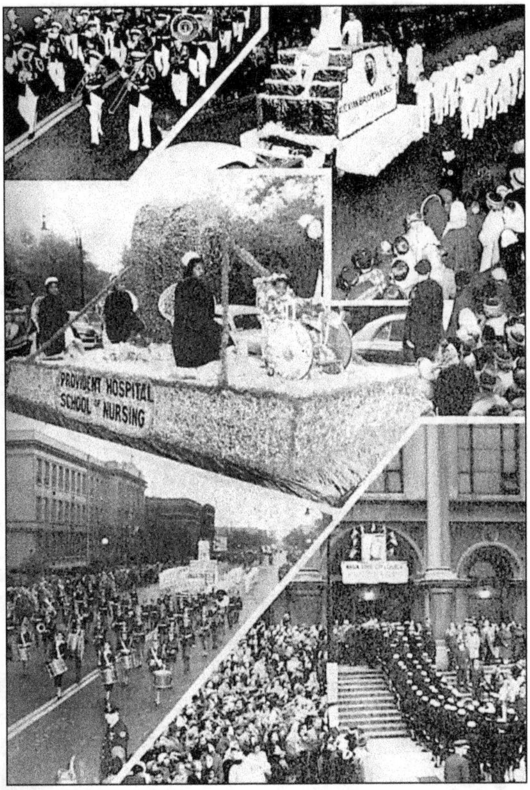

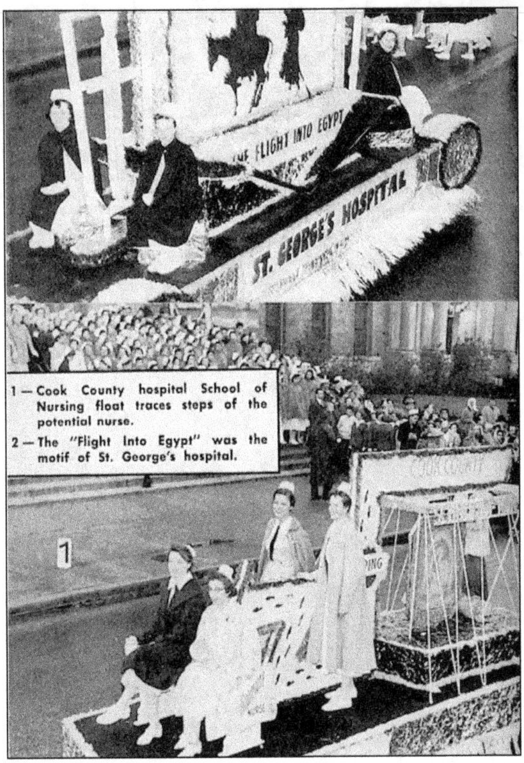

"It was as amazing as watching flowers pop up suddenly after a spring rain. One look and the rain-drenched boulevard was bare of spectators. Another look at a moment after the long day rain stopped and seemingly out of nowhere was thousands of spectators." (John Long, *Novena Notes*, May 31, 1957, 6.) (Photo from *Novena Notes*, May 31, 1957, 4.)

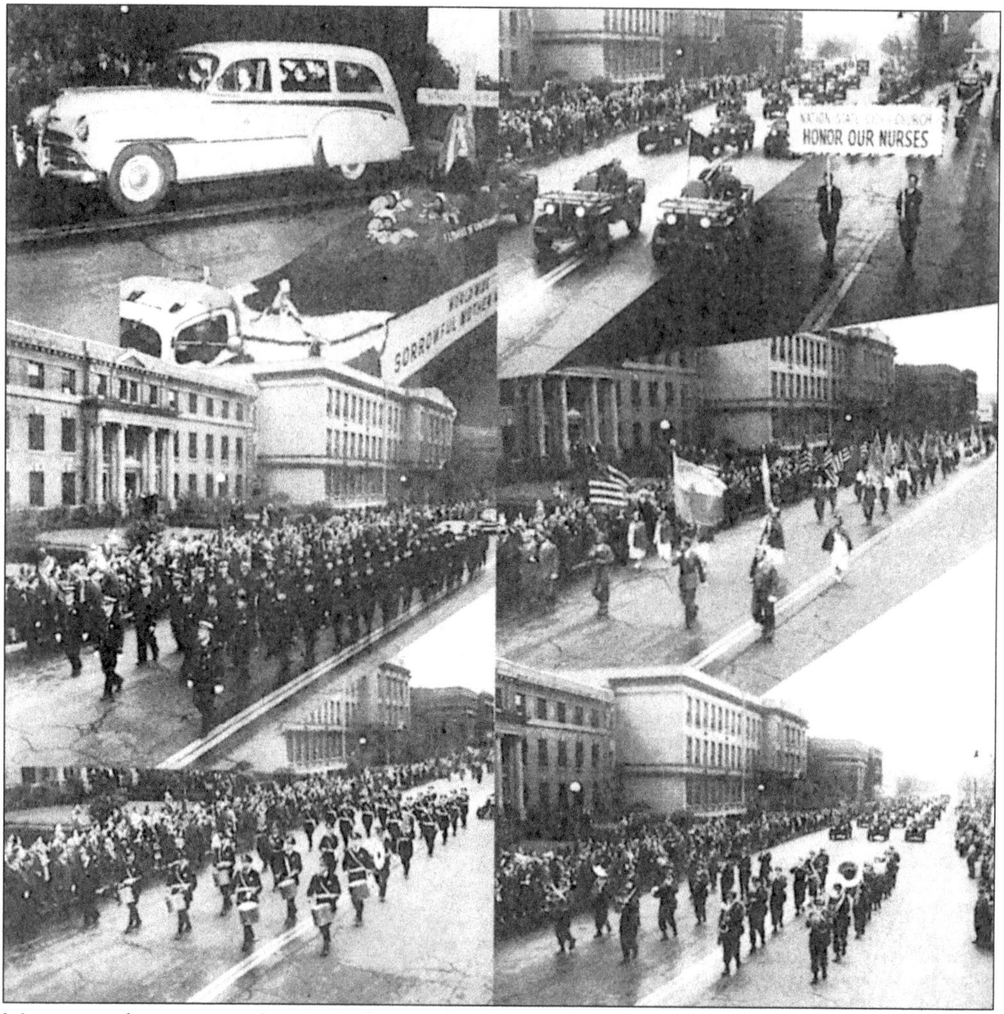

Marines and nursing students march proudly in their blue and whites. (*Novena Notes*, June 13, 1952, 8–9.)

Marching bands are seen here along the parade route. (*Novena Notes*, June 13, 1952, 7.)

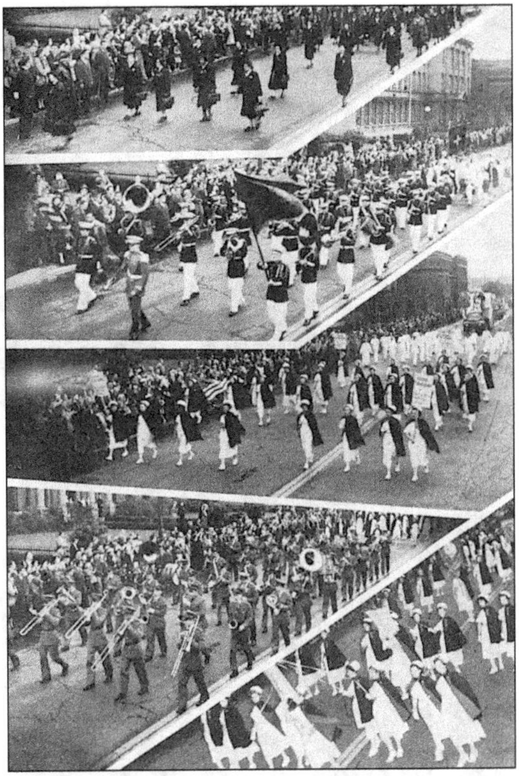

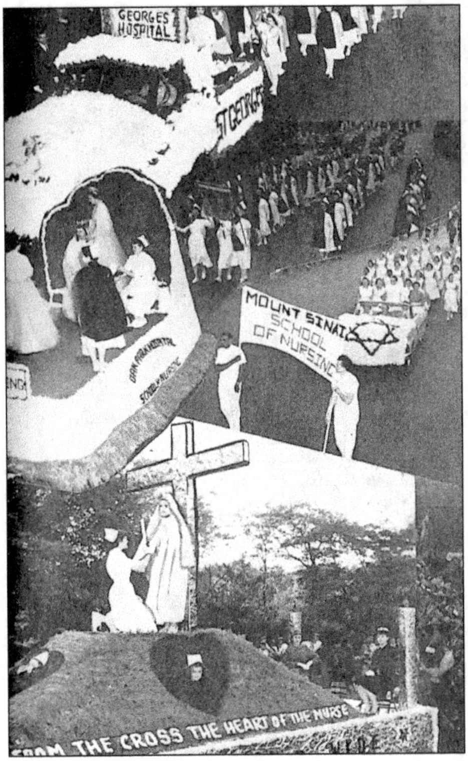

In 1955, nurses and student nurses marched along with the fire and police departments of Chicago. The parade had a new section of 100 international flags. Jackson Boulevard between Albany Avenue and Garfield Park took on a carnival air with red, white, and blue bunting flags. Residents on the route were requested to display a flag. (*Novena Notes*, June 10, 1955, 7.)

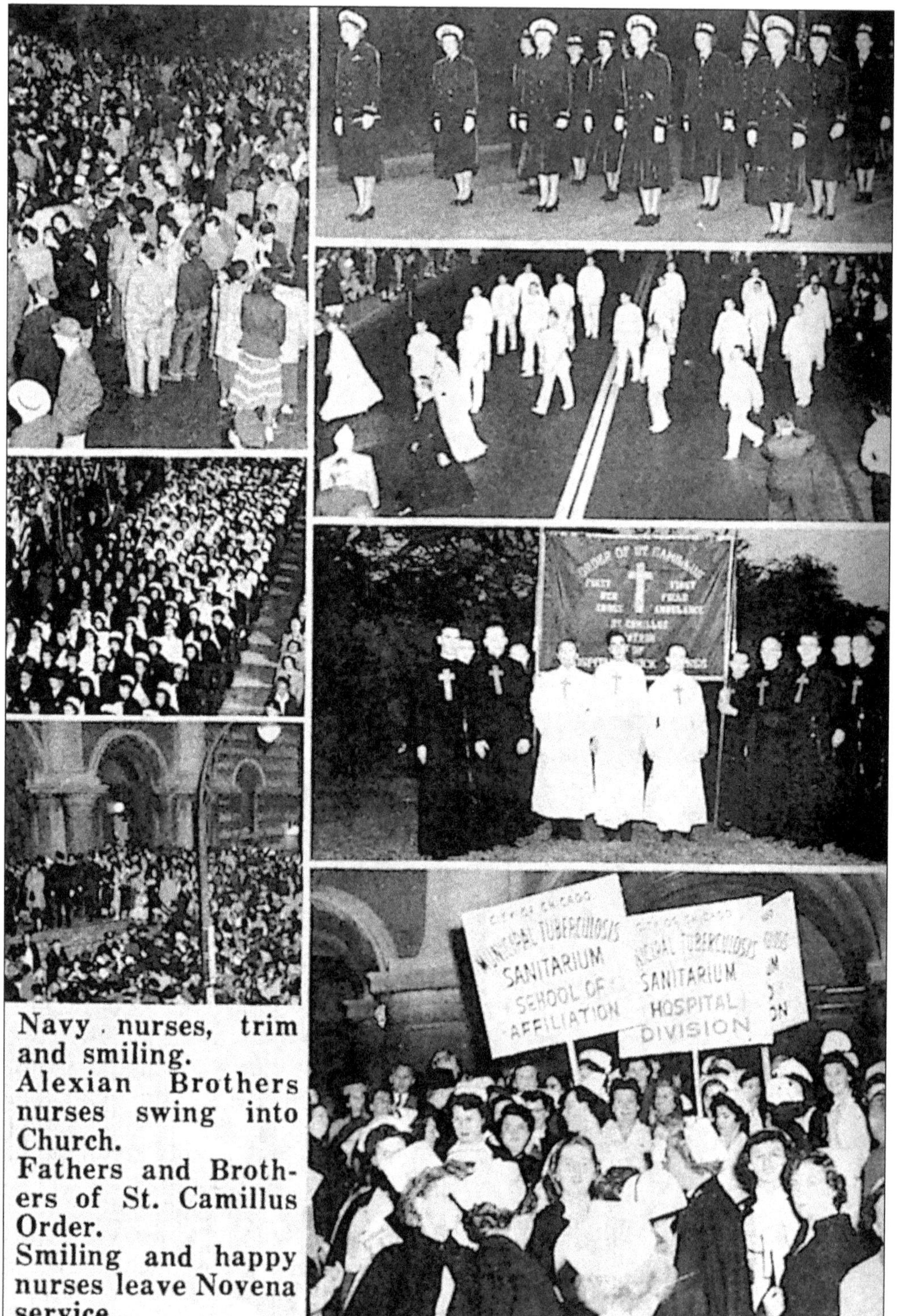

Navy nurses, trim and smiling.
Alexian Brothers nurses swing into Church.
Fathers and Brothers of St. Camillus Order.
Smiling and happy nurses leave Novena service.

Thousands of nurses marched in the parade, captivating spectators. The nurses' joy could be seen as they left the Novena service. (*Novena Notes*, October 6, 1950, 6.)

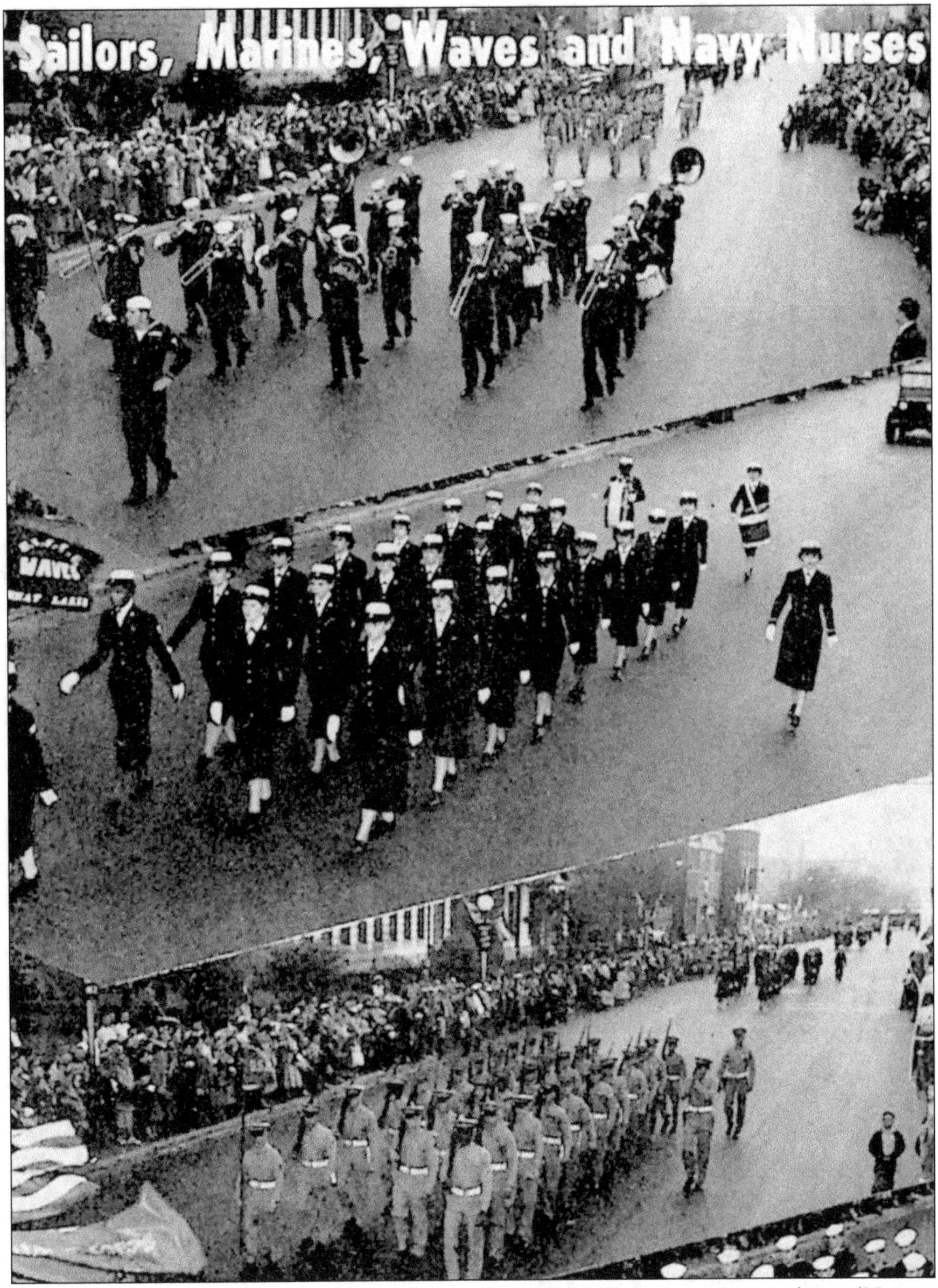

In 1955, the parade included sailors, marines, WAVES, and navy nurses marching. (*Novena Notes*, June 10, 1955, 5.)

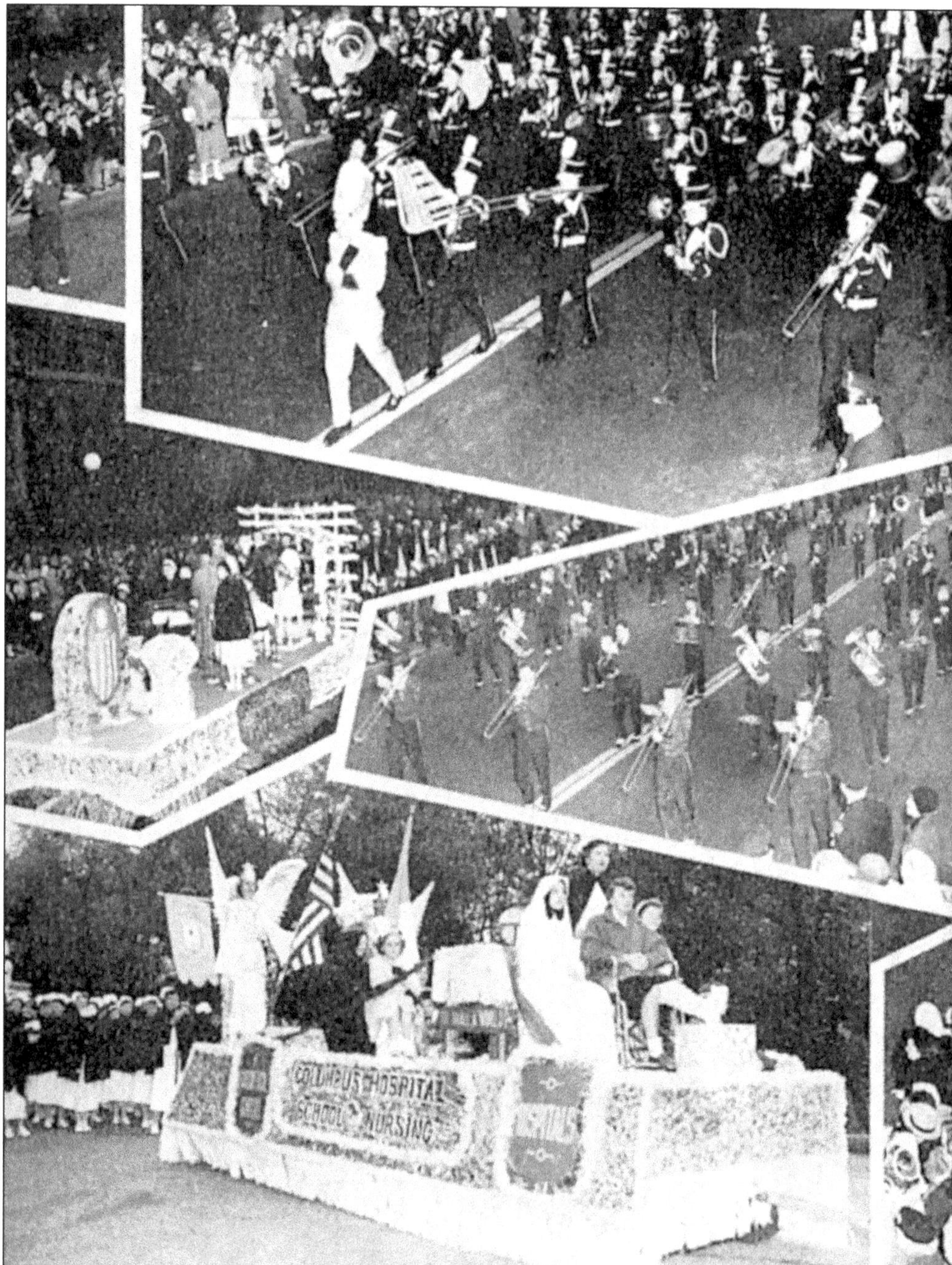

Marching bands in the 1953 Nurses Day Parade are seen here. The final parade in 1958 had over 30 mraching bands. (*Novena Notes*, June 12, 1953, 10.)

Spectators at the parade always applauded the nurses. (*Novena Notes*, June 17, 1955, 2.)

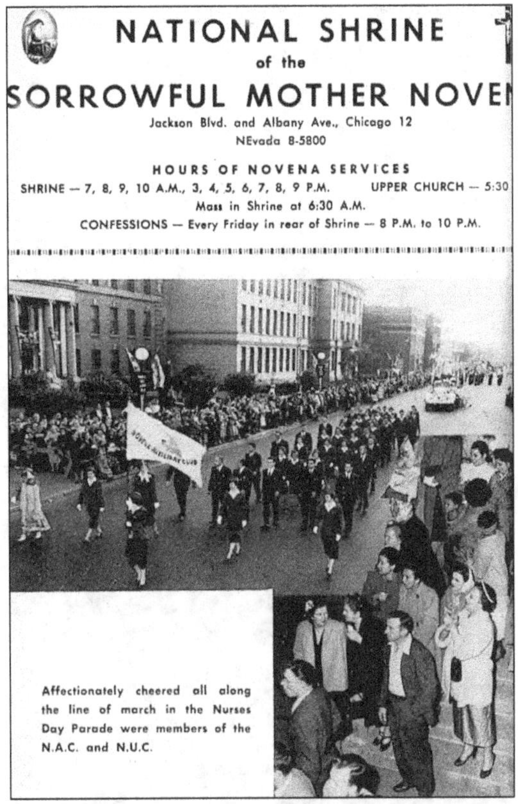

NATIONAL SHRINE

of the

SORROWFUL MOTHER NOVE

Jackson Blvd. and Albany Ave., Chicago 12

NEvada 8-5800

HOURS OF NOVENA SERVICES

SHRINE — 7, 8, 9, 10 A.M., 3, 4, 5, 6, 7, 8, 9 P.M. UPPER CHURCH — 5:30

Mass in Shrine at 6:30 A.M.

CONFESSIONS — Every Friday in rear of Shrine — 8 P.M. to 10 P.M.

Affectionately cheered all along the line of march in the Nurses Day Parade were members of the N.A.C. and N.U.C.

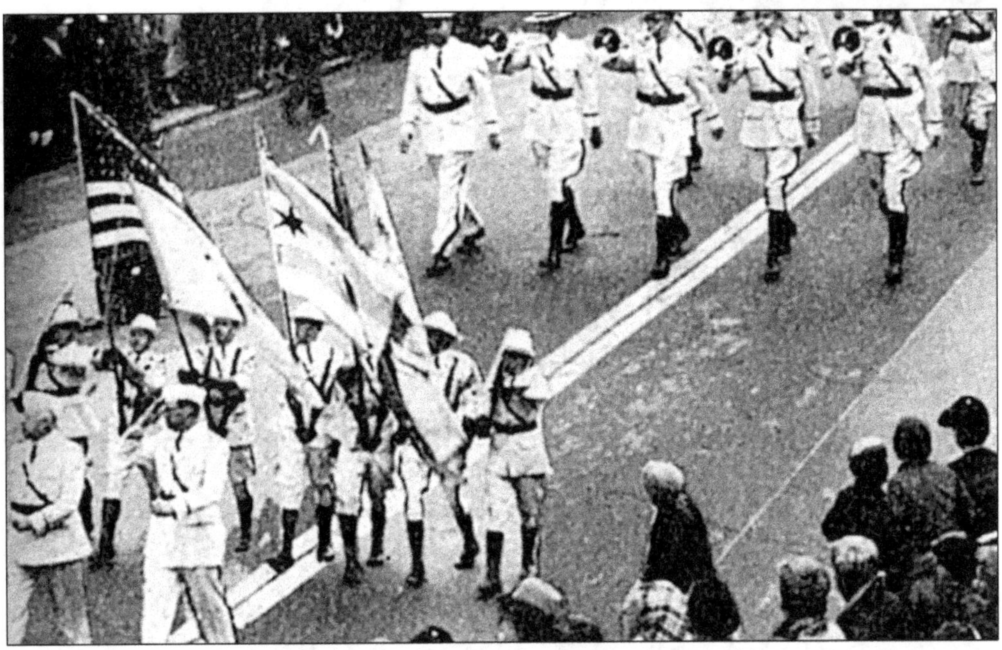

Nurses remembered hearing the bands' music long after the parade was over. Some even remembered the sounds and excitement of the parade when they were caring for their patients. (*Novena Notes*, June 12, 1953, 11.)

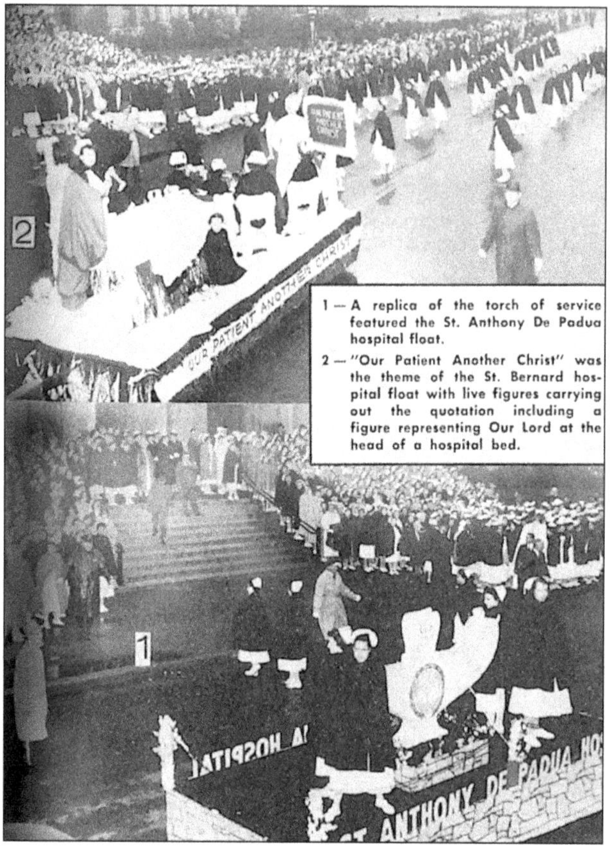

1 — A replica of the torch of service featured the St. Anthony De Padua hospital float.

2 — "Our Patient Another Christ" was the theme of the St. Bernard hospital float with live figures carrying out the quotation including a figure representing Our Lord at the head of a hospital bed.

The 1957 Nurses Day Parade was the first one attended by Major Nicholas Giordano of the U.S. Regular Army. It was reported he could not believe his eyes—2,000 nurses in uniform, 25 floats, 29 bands, and over 75,000 spectators. (*Novena Notes*, May 31, 1957, 7.)

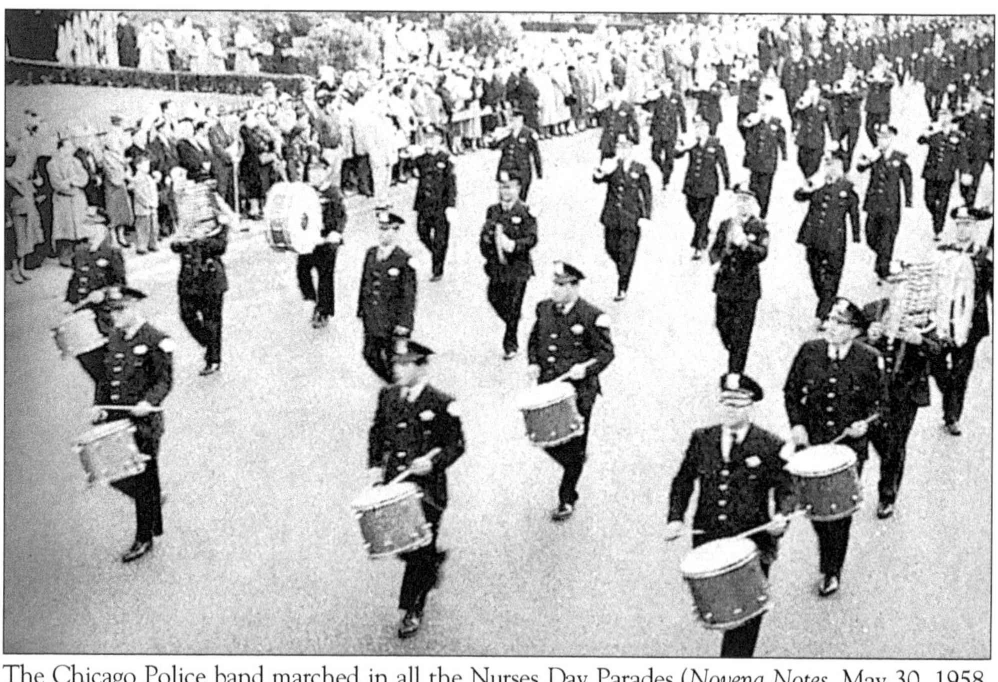

The Chicago Police band marched in all the Nurses Day Parades.(*Novena Notes*, May 30, 1958, 7.)

Colorful floats always stirred the spectators. (*Novena Notes*, Oct, 6, 1950, 10.)

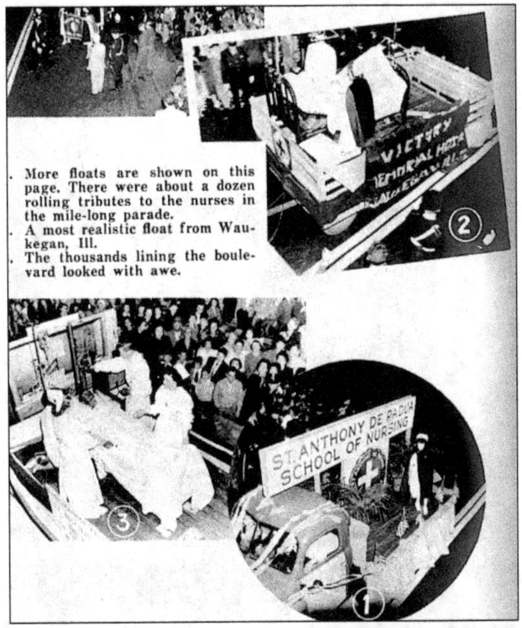

. More floats are shown on this page. There were about a dozen rolling tributes to the nurses in the mile-long parade.
. A most realistic float from Waukegan, Ill.
. The thousands lining the boulevard looked with awe.

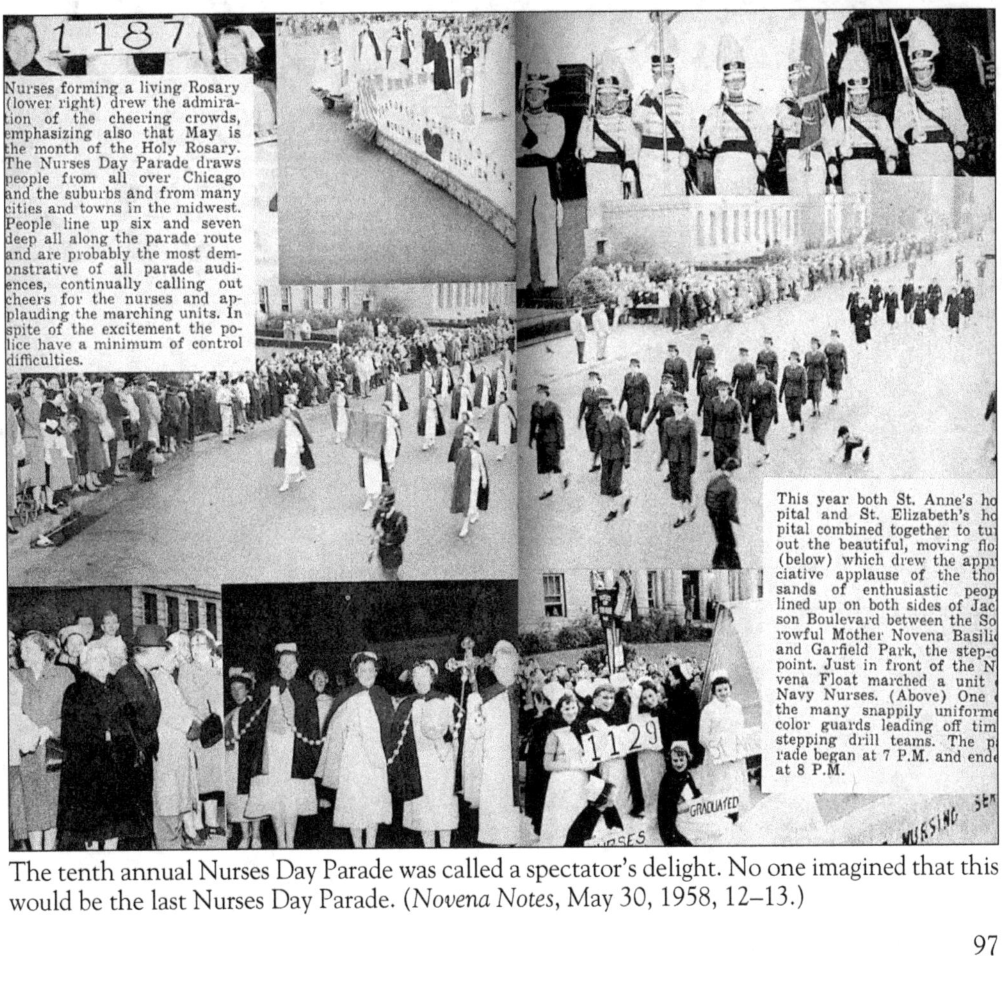

Nurses forming a living Rosary (lower right) drew the admiration of the cheering crowds, emphasizing also that May is the month of the Holy Rosary. The Nurses Day Parade draws people from all over Chicago and the suburbs and from many cities and towns in the midwest. People line up six and seven deep all along the parade route and are probably the most demonstrative of all parade audiences, continually calling out cheers for the nurses and applauding the marching units. In spite of the excitement the police have a minimum of control difficulties.

This year both St. Anne's ho pital and St. Elizabeth's ho pital combined together to tu out the beautiful, moving flo (below) which drew the appr ciative applause of the tho sands of enthusiastic peop lined up on both sides of Jac son Boulevard between the So rowful Mother Novena Basili and Garfield Park, the step-o point. Just in front of the N vena Float marched a unit Navy Nurses. (Above) One the many snappily uniform color guards leading off tim stepping drill teams. The p rade began at 7 P.M. and end at 8 P.M.

The tenth annual Nurses Day Parade was called a spectator's delight. No one imagined that this would be the last Nurses Day Parade. (*Novena Notes*, May 30, 1958, 12–13.)

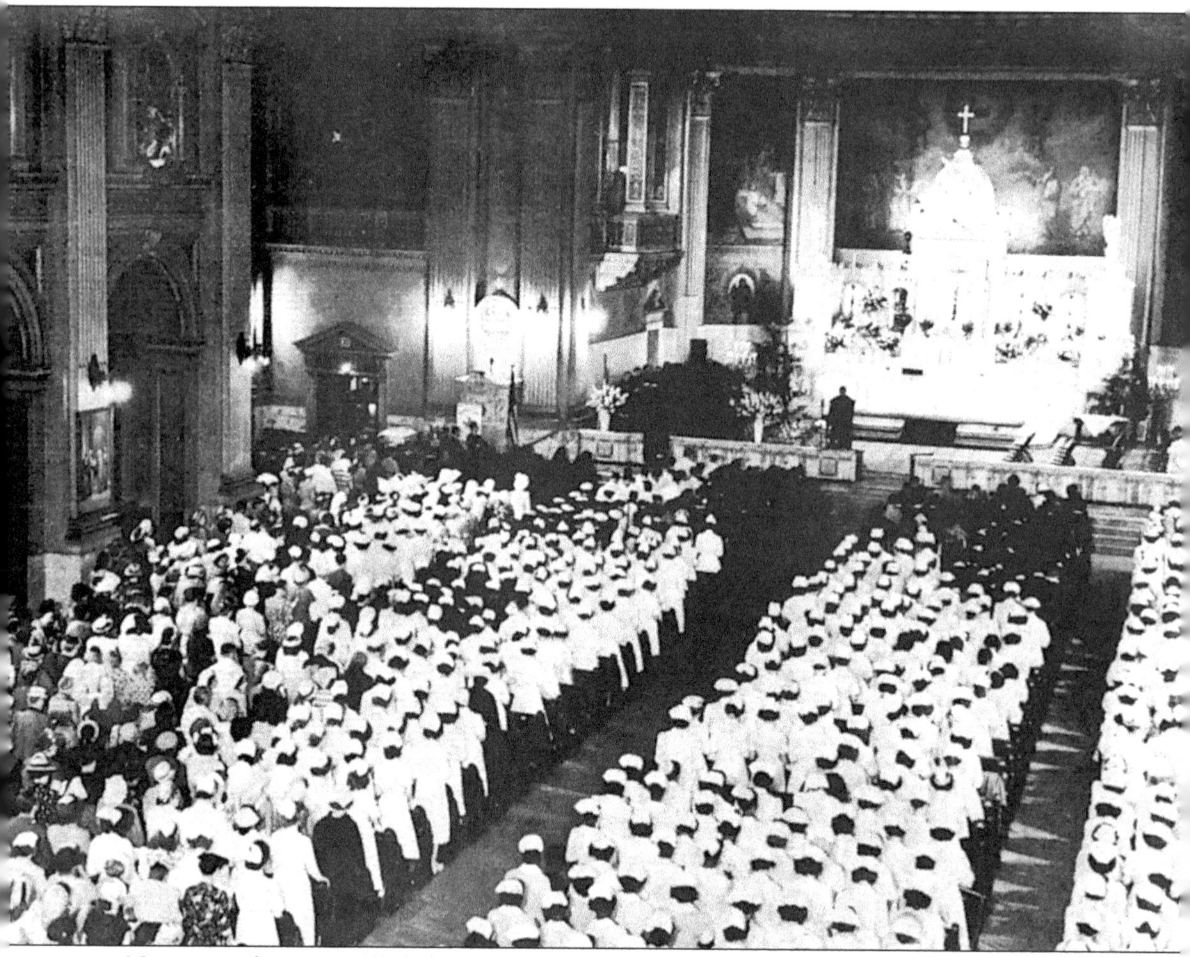

Nurses in white caps filled the National Shrine in 1948 as a prelude to the parade in 1949. (*Novena Notes*, August 5, 1949, back cover.)

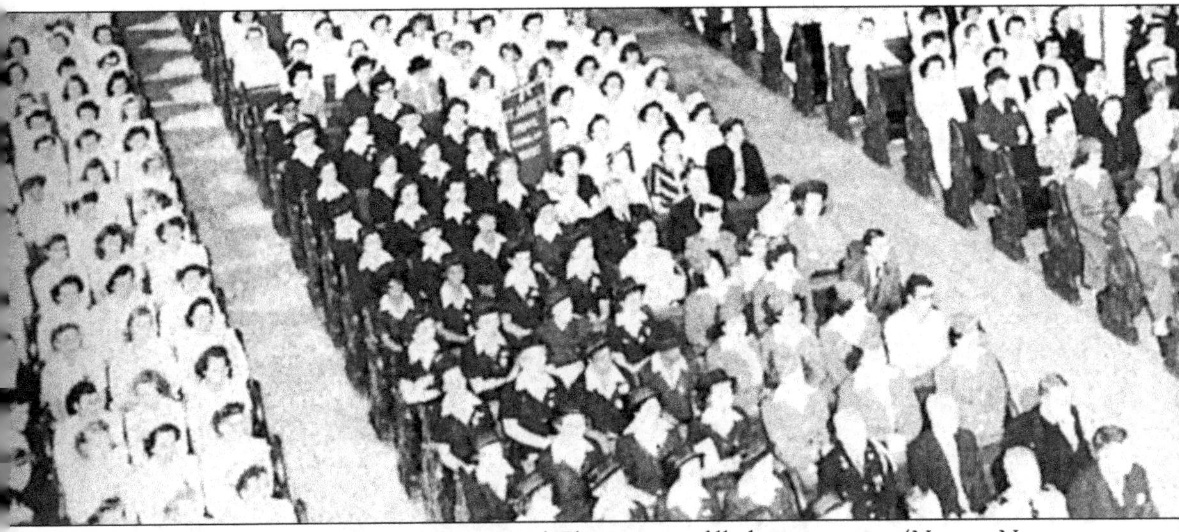

The upper and lower levels of the National Shrine were filled to capacity. (*Novena Notes*, August 5, 1949, 7.)

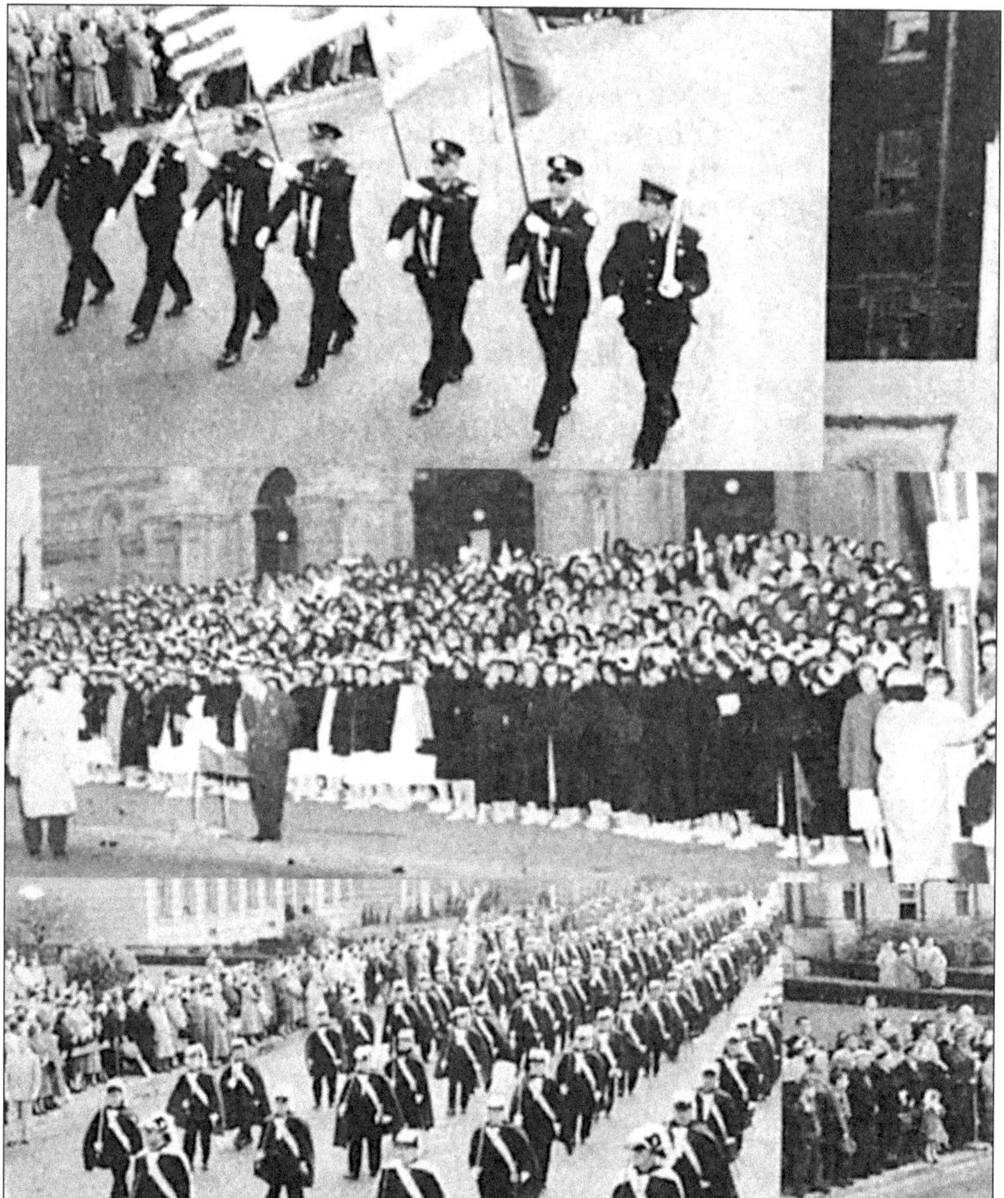

City, state, and national officials all celebrated the work of nurses by participating in the parade in full uniform. (*Novena Notes*, May 30, 1958, 7.)

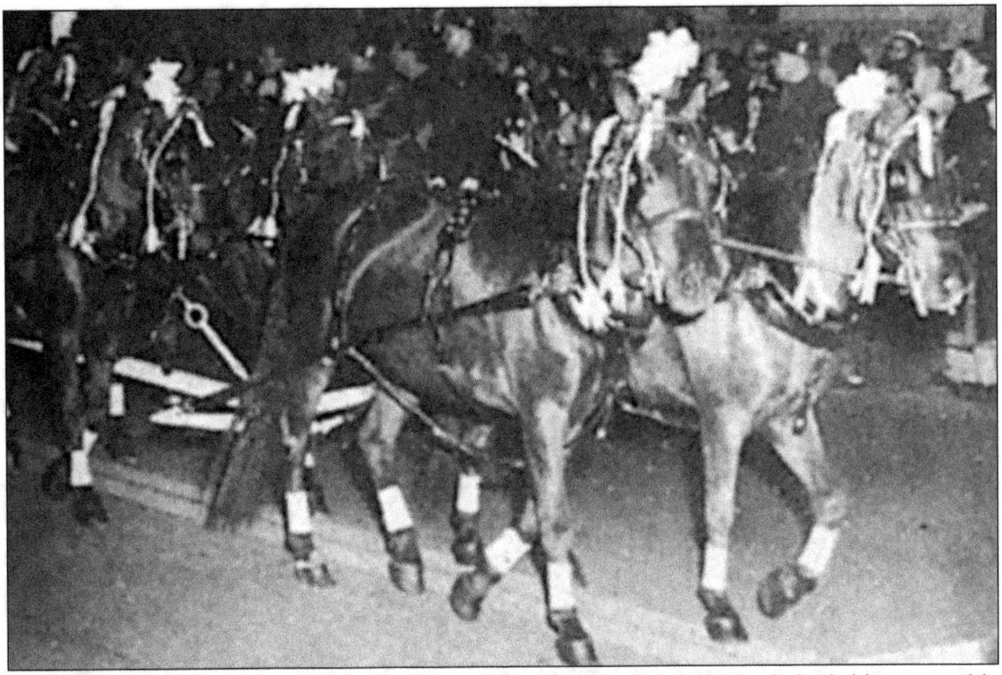

The 1956 parade was the first in which the Shriners' Hospital for Crippled Children was able to participate. They had a float, a pony-drawn carriage, the Black Horse Troop with 60 men on horseback, and, of course, a unit of marching nurses. (*Novena Notes*, June 8, 1956, 5.)

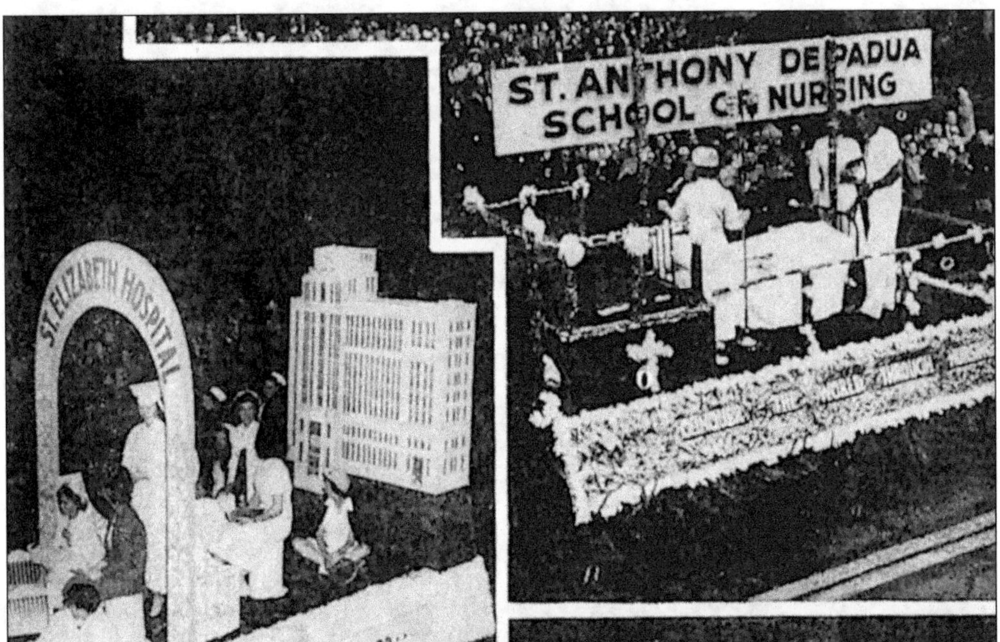

Floats were tributes to nursing schools in the 1952 parade, "Steps to Nurse Hood." (*Novena Notes*, June 13, 1952, back cover.)

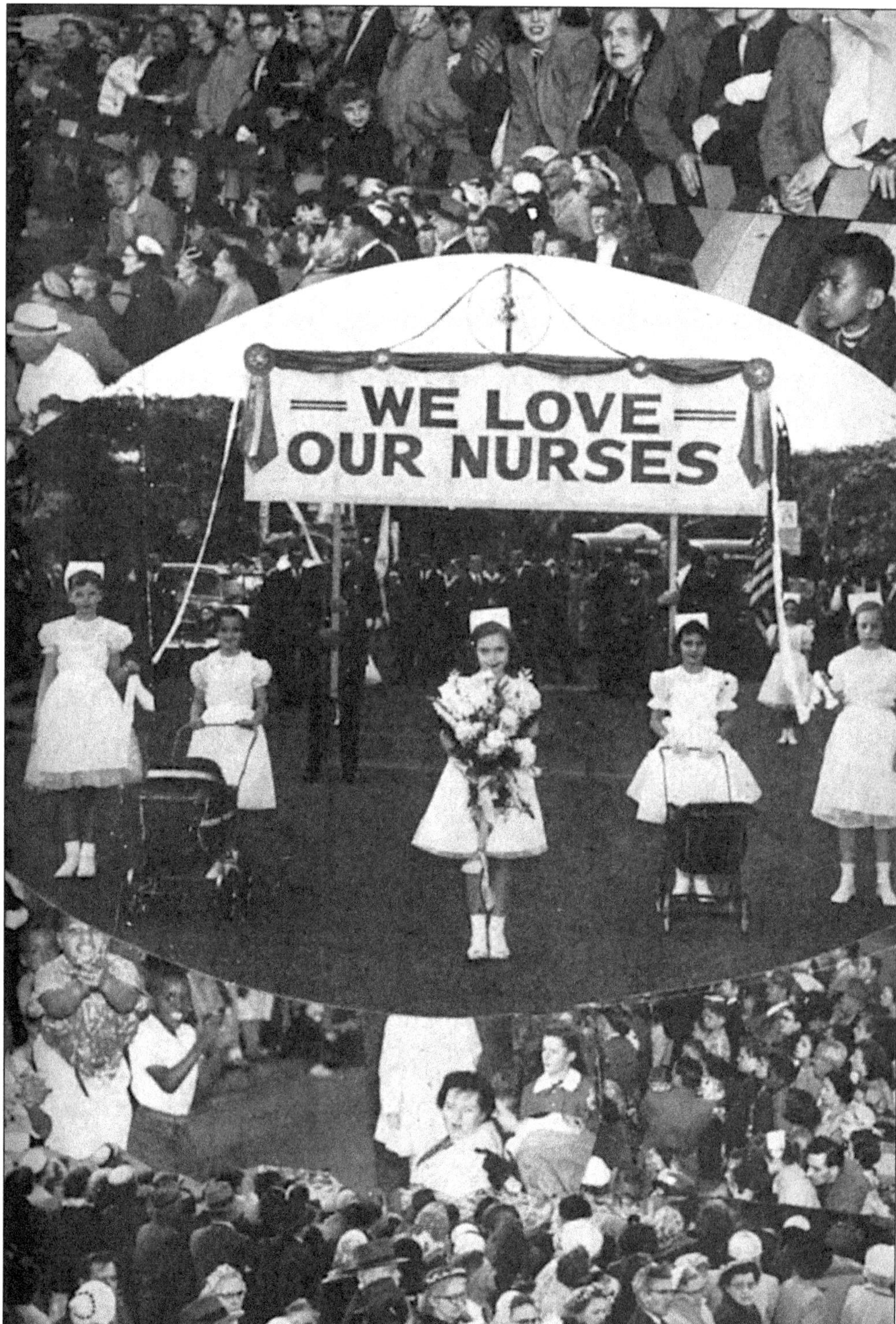

All the parades reinforced an appreciation for the work of nurses. (*Novena Notes*, June 10, 1955, cover.)

Five

Nurses Remember . . . The Parade

The Nurses Day Parade was last held in the city of Chicago almost 50 years ago. Nurses who marched in the parade are now in their sixties, seventies, or older. Nurses, both then and now, truly appreciated the public honor given to them in the parade.

Although the parade only lasted a decade and was almost 50 years ago, the sentiments, meaning, and memories of the parade are still vibrant and alive in the hearts and minds of those nurses who participated.

Constance L. Earle reported that she recently attended her class of 1955 St. Anne's Nursing School reunion. At the reunion she and her classmates fondly reminisced about the Nurses Day Parade. Another nurse remembers her sadness in 1959 when there was not an invitation for her nursing school to attend the parade; she realized that there was not going to be a Nurses Day Parade that year; she never anticipated that there would never be another.

Loretta Mostaccio was one of 2,000 nurses who marched in the Nurses Day Parade. She lives in Elmwood Park and recalls that marching in the parade was "quite an honor." Loretta was a student at St. Anne's Hospital when she marched in the parade in the early 1950s. "I remember being very excited about it," says Mostaccio. "I remember making this big globe out of papier-mâché. Our float was the Queen of Nations float. We had flags of all kinds." Loretta marched in the parade that honored nurses of different nationalities.

Janet Hantsch, R.N., of Lisle, a 1958 graduate of St. Xavier University School of Nursing, marched in the 1956 parade. "I remember how proud we were to be included in this event," she says. "As I recall, we marched from Garfield Park to Our Lady of Sorrows Basilica where a ceremony was held."

"I entered Saint Margaret Hospital School of Nursing in Hammond, Indiana in September 1957; and, if I am not mistaken, it may have been in 1958 when our school was invited to march in Nurses Day Parade," says Nancy Kolinski, R.N. "I shall always remember it. It was breathtaking. As we marched into the church, which was lit only with candles, each nurse held a lighted candle. As we all sang 'Ave, Ave, Maria,' we raised our candles up as we went to our seats. One of my classmates, who was not a Catholic, sat in the pew and just cried. When we asked why she was crying, she said she had never seen anything so beautiful with all of us in uniform."

Marybeth Young, R.N., of Chicago, says she was with the float thanking Salk for his discovery. "As a 1955 graduate of St. Elizabeth's Hospital School of Nursing, I have fond memories of the parade," she says. "We had chartered buses to take us to Jackson Boulevard where each group connected with floats assembled at the various schools and agencies."

Chicago's Nurses Day Parade ended abruptly in 1958 when Brissette left as the national Novena director of the Basilica and was assigned a different role by the Servite Order. After 1958, there was no further mention of the parade in *Novena Notes* or newspapers.

Nursing continues to be an undermanned profession made up of noble and caring men and women. What is a good nurse? Perhaps a good nurse can still be described as it was in 1956. "A good nurse wears a cool brow and carries a candle in [his or her] heart. A good nurse's morals are as clean as the cap [he or she] wears. A good nurse rarely shows [he or she] is tired, yet their manner gives rest to the weary. A good nurse is serene, though [he or she] may be battling butterflies inside. A good nurse has a sense of humor. A good nurse is a gift God gives his sick children." (Marguerite Ratty Brophy, *Novena Notes*, May 18, 1956, 10.)

Barbara Feltman was Barbara Buck in 1954, a junior student nurse at St. Francis Nursing School in Evanston. She remembers marching in the Nurses Day Parade. She marched in a grey cape with red lining. The march took her down Jackson Boulevard to Our Lady of Sorrows' candlelit church where she renewed her nursing vows. Barbara, nearly 50 years later, not only remembers the parade but remembers her emotions. She was proud to be a nurse, honored to be in the parade and felt important and elegant as she marched down Jackson Boulevard.

Some nurses of today may have never known about the parade, other nurses may have left behind the faded memories of the Nurses Day Parade. However, those who participated in the parade will never forget the honor, respect, vitality, and values of nurses, all publicly recognized in their "day of glory" during the decade of the Nurses Day Parade.

(Excerpts modified with permission from J. Boivin, "Chicago Nurses' Parade," *Nursing Spectrum*, January 2004.)

Souvenir of the

SEVENTH ANNUAL NURSES DAY PARADE

MAY 20, 1955

Sponsored by the

SORROWFUL MOTHER NOVENA

"And thy own soul a sword shall pierce, that out of many hearts thoughts may be revealed."

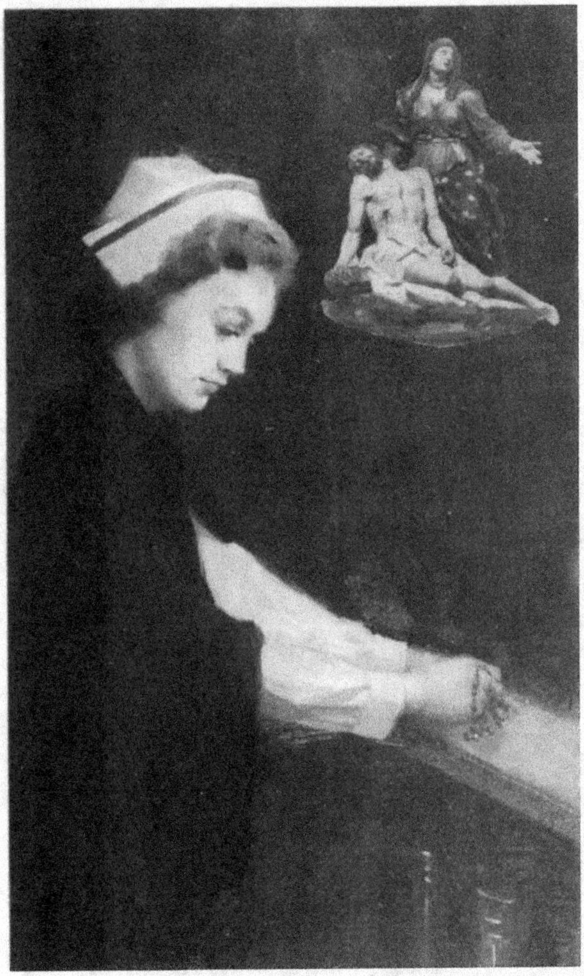

EVERY FRIDAY IS NOVENA DAY

Some of the hospitals, schools of nurses, newspapers, and merchants who participated in a decade of the Nurses Day Parade are no longer in existence. However, those who did participate in the parade have the memories of the parade in their hearts and minds.

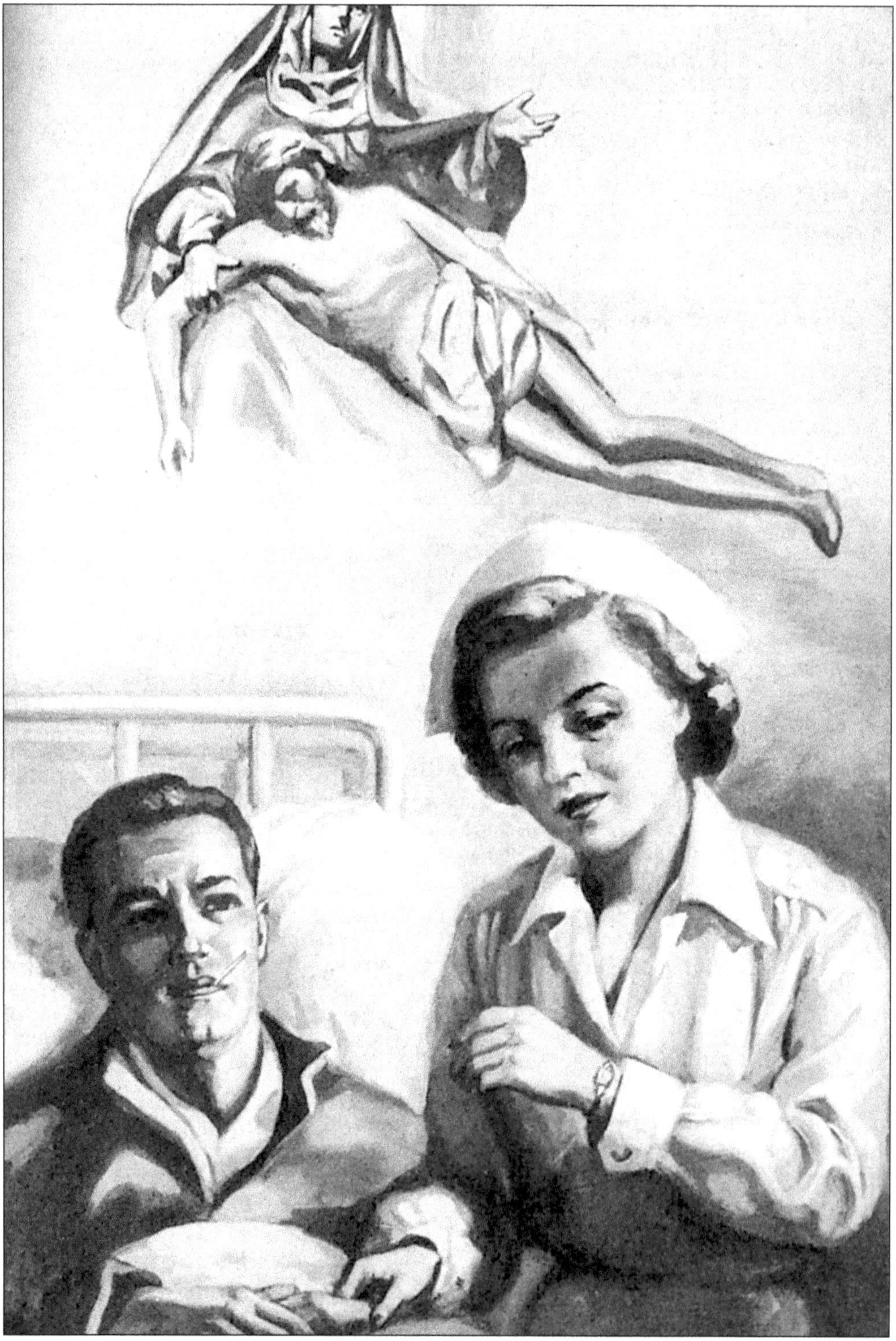

This cover of the *Novena Notes* from May 18, 1956 was an original drawing by Edna Weber, a Chicago artist. The Novena service after the parade focused on the individual qualities of a nurse.

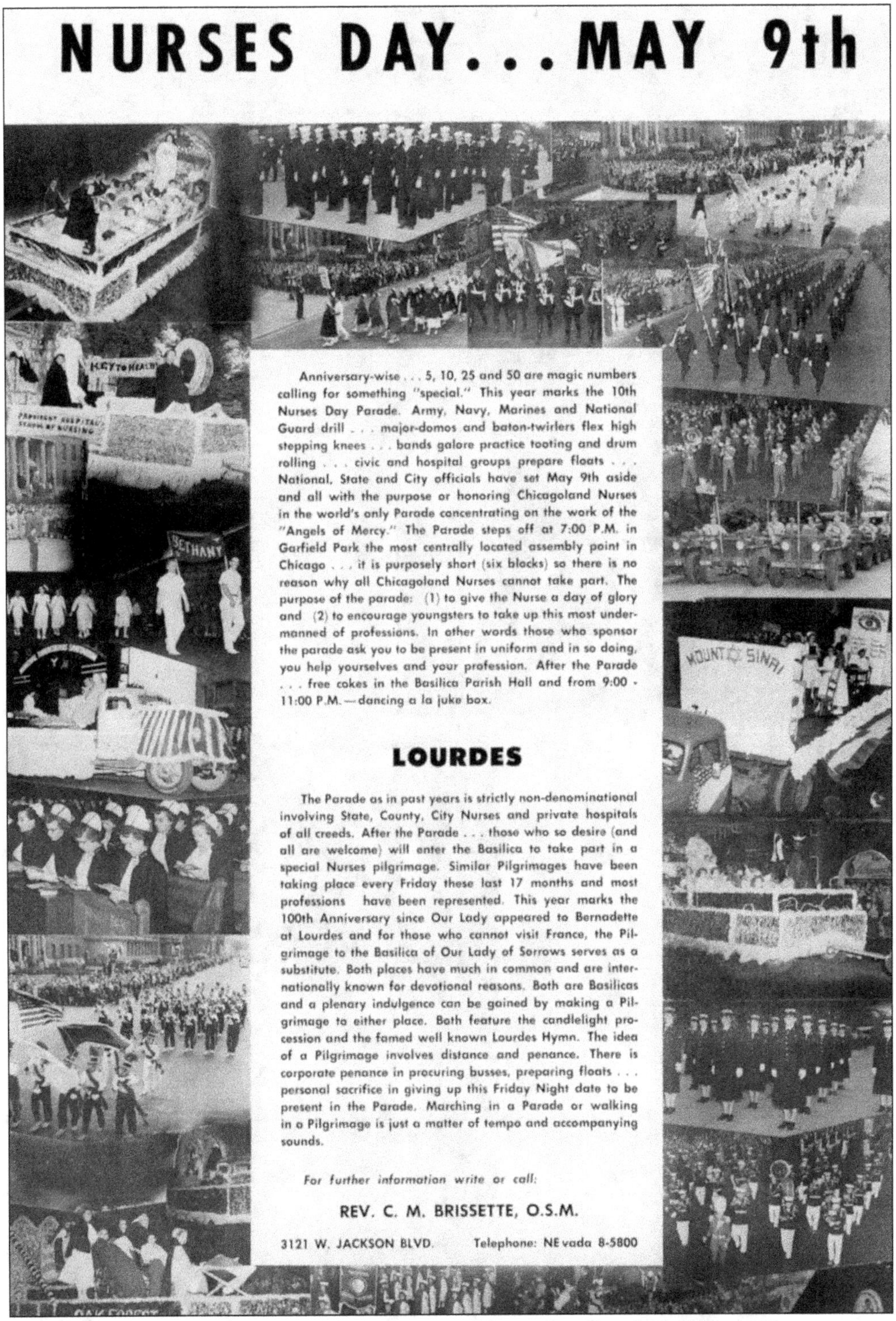
NURSES DAY...MAY 9th
Anniversary-wise . . . 5, 10, 25 and 50 are magic numbers calling for something "special." This year marks the 10th Nurses Day Parade. Army, Navy, Marines and National Guard drill . . . major-domos and baton-twirlers flex high stepping knees . . . bands galore practice tooting and drum rolling . . . civic and hospital groups prepare floats . . . National, State and City officials have set May 9th aside and all with the purpose or honoring Chicagoland Nurses in the world's only Parade concentrating on the work of the "Angels of Mercy." The Parade steps off at 7:00 P.M. in Garfield Park the most centrally located assembly point in Chicago . . . it is purposely short (six blocks) so there is no reason why all Chicagoland Nurses cannot take part. The purpose of the parade: (1) to give the Nurse a day of glory and (2) to encourage youngsters to take up this most undermanned of professions. In other words those who sponsor the parade ask you to be present in uniform and in so doing, you help yourselves and your profession. After the Parade . . . free cokes in the Basilica Parish Hall and from 9:00 - 11:00 P.M.—dancing a la juke box.
LOURDES
The Parade as in past years is strictly non-denominational involving State, County, City Nurses and private hospitals of all creeds. After the Parade . . . those who so desire (and all are welcome) will enter the Basilica to take part in a special Nurses pilgrimage. Similar Pilgrimages have been taking place every Friday these last 17 months and most professions have been represented. This year marks the 100th Anniversary since Our Lady appeared to Bernadette at Lourdes and for those who cannot visit France, the Pilgrimage to the Basilica of Our Lady of Sorrows serves as a substitute. Both places have much in common and are internationally known for devotional reasons. Both are Basilicas and a plenary indulgence can be gained by making a Pilgrimage to either place. Both feature the candlelight procession and the famed well known Lourdes Hymn. The idea of a Pilgrimage involves distance and penance. There is corporate penance in procuring busses, preparing floats . . . personal sacrifice in giving up this Friday Night date to be present in the Parade. Marching in a Parade or walking in a Pilgrimage is just a matter of tempo and accompanying sounds.
For further information write or call:
REV. C. M. BRISSETTE, O.S.M.
3121 W. JACKSON BLVD.
Telephone: NEvada 8-5800
BETHANY
MOUNT SINAI

This is the poster for Chicago's 10th Anniversary Nurses Day Parade, held in 1958.

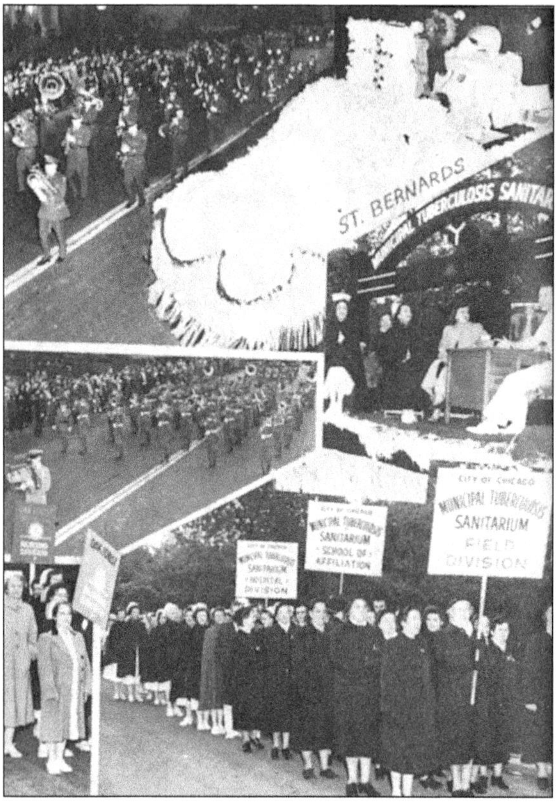

County, city, and private hospital nurses, along with precision drill teams, massed flags holders, and Catholic War Vets all marched or had floats in the 1953 Nurses Day Parade (*Novena Notes*, June 12, 1953, 12.)

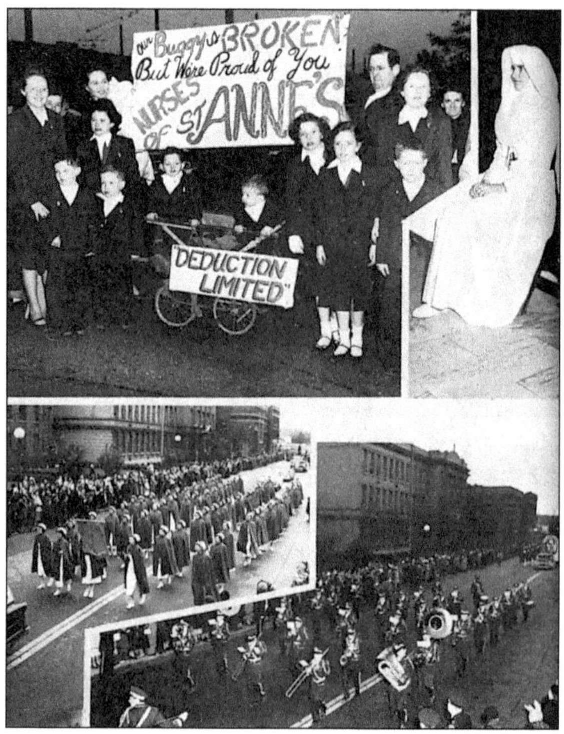

The newspapers estimated that, in 1953, 50,000 to 100,000 spectators lined the streets to watch the Nurses Day Parade. The Brennan children, all born at St. Anne's Hospital, were among these spectators. (*Novena Notes*, June 12, 1953, 16.)

Nurses appreciated the parade, as demonstrated in this letter: "On behalf of the M.T.S. Field Nurses of Stock Yards Clinic, who attended the Nurses Day Parade, we wish to thank you most heartily for your praiseworthy achievements in giving the high mark of honor to nurses," signed by Catherine L. Bell, R.N., Elizabeth Zieske, R.N., Gertrude Killeen, R.N., and Margaret Lynch, R.N. (*Novena Notes*, June 19, 1953, 13.)

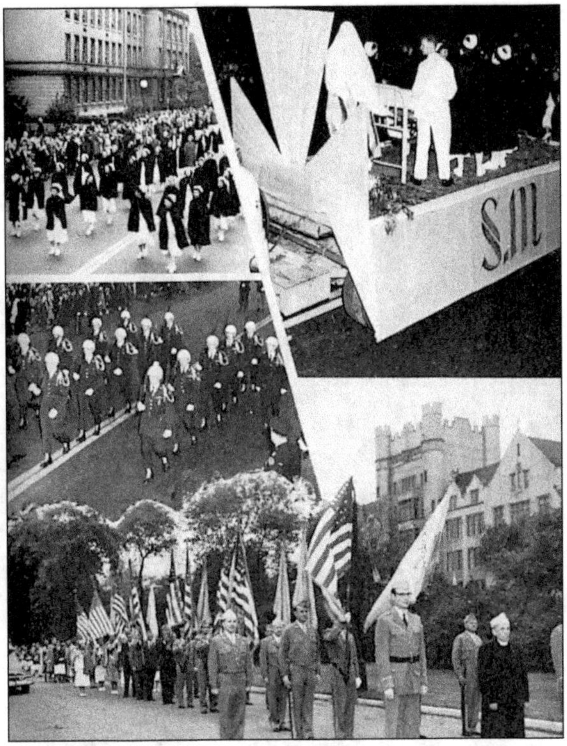

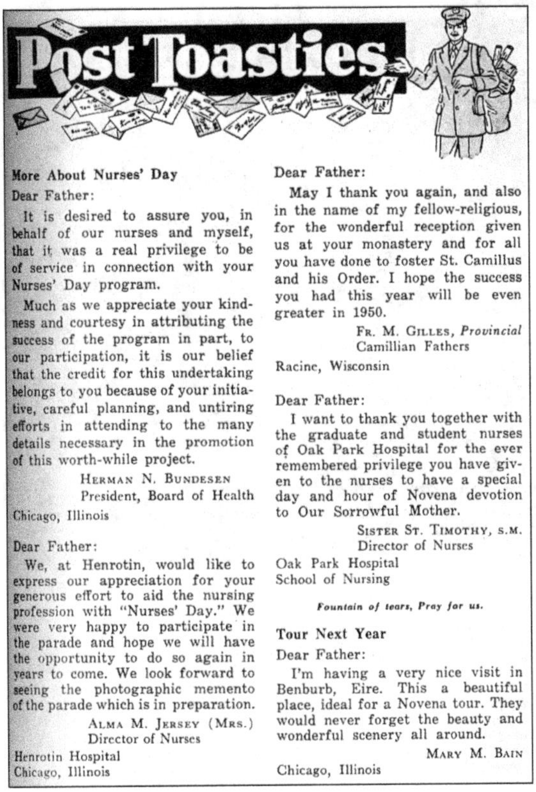

Post Toasties

More About Nurses' Day

Dear Father:

It is desired to assure you, in behalf of our nurses and myself, that it was a real privilege to be of service in connection with your Nurses' Day program.

Much as we appreciate your kindness and courtesy in attributing the success of the program in part, to our participation, it is our belief that the credit for this undertaking belongs to you because of your initiative, careful planning, and untiring efforts in attending to the many details necessary in the promotion of this worth-while project.

HERMAN N. BUNDESEN
President, Board of Health

Chicago, Illinois

Dear Father:

We, at Henrotin, would like to express our appreciation for your generous effort to aid the nursing profession with "Nurses' Day." We were very happy to participate in the parade and hope we will have the opportunity to do so again in years to come. We look forward to seeing the photographic memento of the parade which is in preparation.

ALMA M. JERSEY (MRS.)
Director of Nurses

Henrotin Hospital
Chicago, Illinois

Dear Father:

May I thank you again, and also in the name of my fellow-religious, for the wonderful reception given us at your monastery and for all you have done to foster St. Camillus and his Order. I hope the success you had this year will be even greater in 1950.

FR. M. GILLES, *Provincial*
Camillian Fathers

Racine, Wisconsin

Dear Father:

I want to thank you together with the graduate and student nurses of Oak Park Hospital for the ever remembered privilege you have given to the nurses to have a special day and hour of Novena devotion to Our Sorrowful Mother.

SISTER ST. TIMOTHY, S.M.
Director of Nurses

Oak Park Hospital
School of Nursing

Fountain of tears, Pray for us.

Tour Next Year

Dear Father:

I'm having a very nice visit in Benburb, Eire. This a beautiful place, ideal for a Novena tour. They would never forget the beauty and wonderful scenery all around.

MARY M. BAIN

Chicago, Illinois

The parade was appreciated by all, as witnessed in these "Post Toasties" letters. (*Novena Notes*, Aug. 26, 1949, 5.)

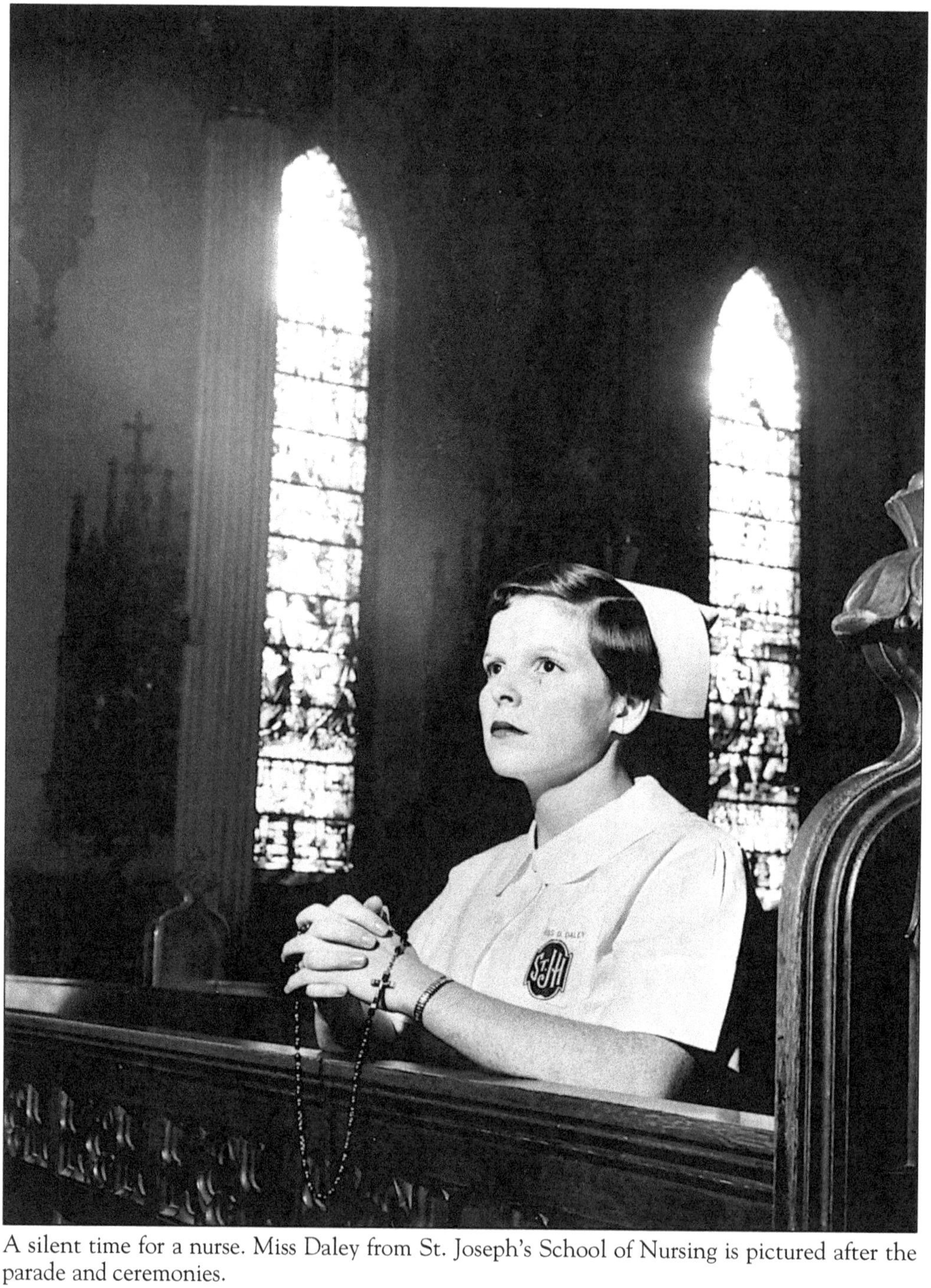

A silent time for a nurse. Miss Daley from St. Joseph's School of Nursing is pictured after the parade and ceremonies.

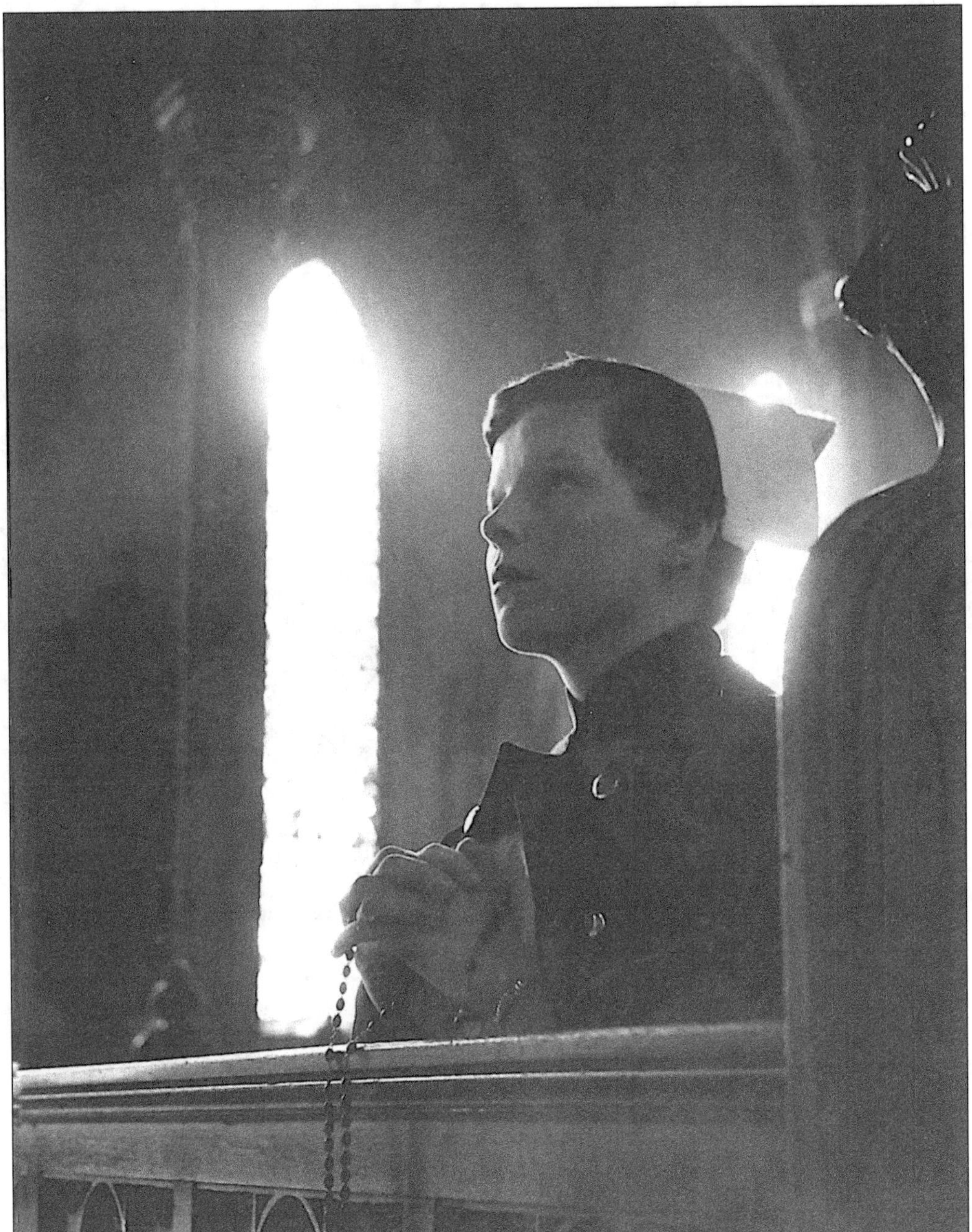

A student nurse reflecting after the parade and ceremonies.

Do You Remember the Chicago Nurses Parade?

Nursing Spectrum is looking for nurses who participated in or remember the Chicago Nurses Parade, which was held annually between 1948 and 1958.

The parade is a long-lost piece of Chicago nursing history recently rediscovered with the help of Rev. Conrad Borntrager, who marched in the parade's band and who is a historian for the Servants of Mary Servists.

The parade was organized by Our Lady of Sorrow Church at 3121 West Jackson Avenue and was attended by thousands of nurses and community members. The parade also featured floats sponsored by local hospitals and marching bands.

If you have information about the parade, please call Janet Boivin, RN, editorial director, at 847/839-1700 or e-mail her at jboivin@nursingspectrum.com.

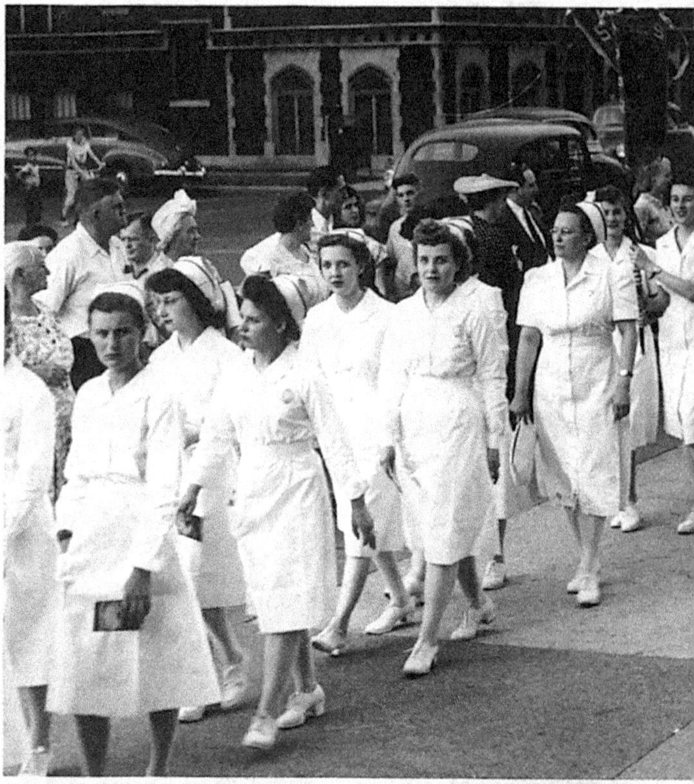

Nurses march in the first Nurses Parade in 1948 Chi
Photo courtesy of Our Lady of Sorrow Church.

Janet Boivin wanted to write an article that would reflect the true stories of nurses who participated in the parade. Prior to writing the article, Janet called for testimony, requesting nurses to tell their stories of the parade. (*Nursing Spectrum*, November 2003.)

Father Conrad Borntrager, religious order of the Servants of Mary (Servites), is Provincial Archivist at Our Lady of Sorrows Basilica. He meticulously preserved the history of the parade. Father Conrad also marched in several in several of the parades as a member of the St. Philip High School band. Father Conrad assisted in editing this book and is extremely pleased that the parade is now remembered, visible for all to share. (Photo courtesy of *Nursing Spectrum*.)

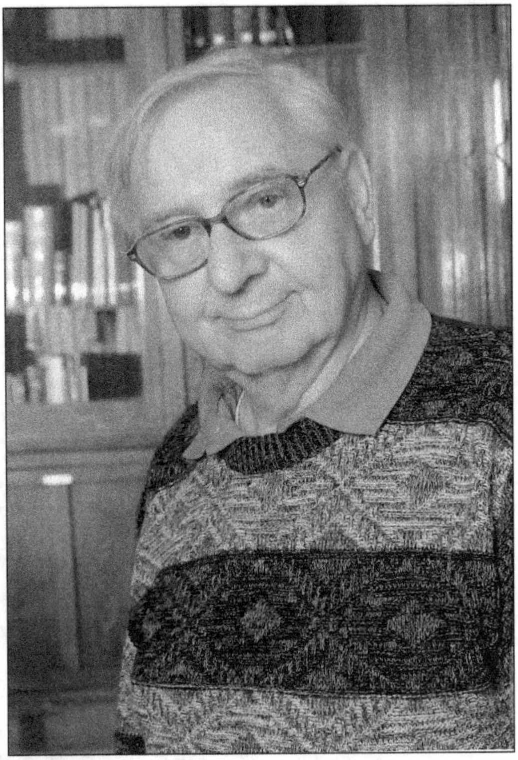

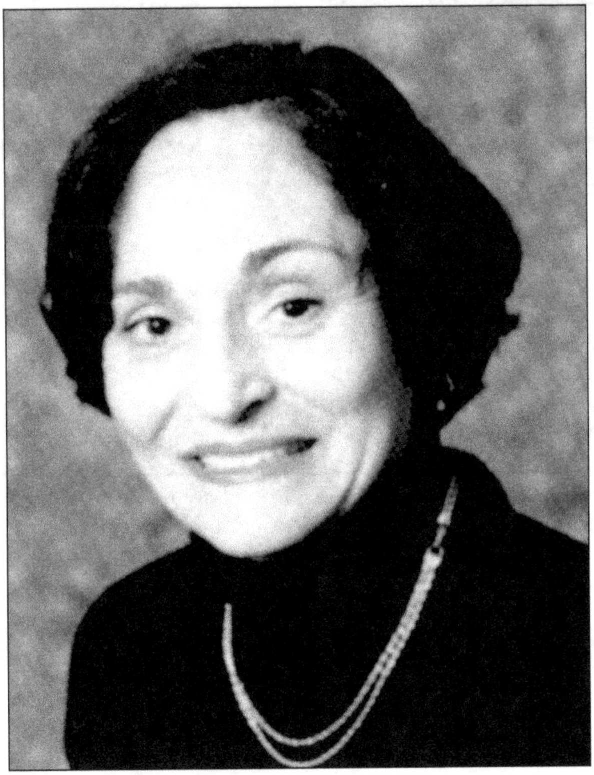

Janet Boivin, R.N., editorial director for the greater Chicago/tri-state *Nursing Spectrum*, saw the value in nurses remembering and sharing their experiences of participating in the Nurses Day Parade. (Photo courtesy of *Nursing Spectrum*.)

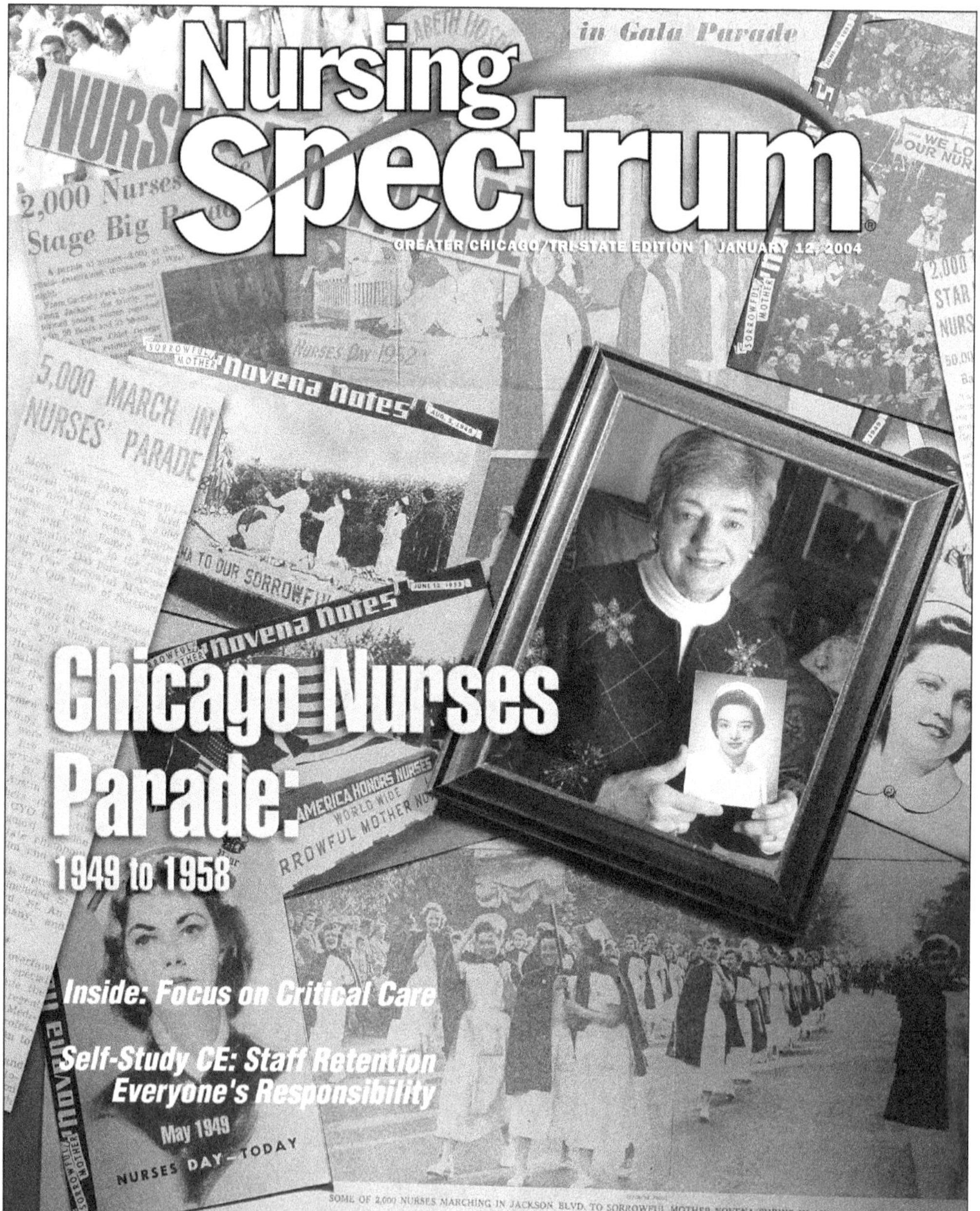

Janet Boivin wrote the first article in over 45 years about the Nurses Day Parade. She provided the first forum for nurses to share their memories of the parade. (Cover of *Nursing Spectrum*, January 2004.)

Loretta Mostaccio, R.N., recalls marching in the nurses' parade as "quite an honor." She marched in the early 1950s as a St. Anne's student nurse. When St. Anne's had a float of the globe, Loretta was on a pedestal over the globe dressed as the Virgin Mary. (Janet Boivin, "Chicago Nurses' Parade," *Nursing Spectrum*, January 2004; photo courtesy of *Nursing Spectrum*.)

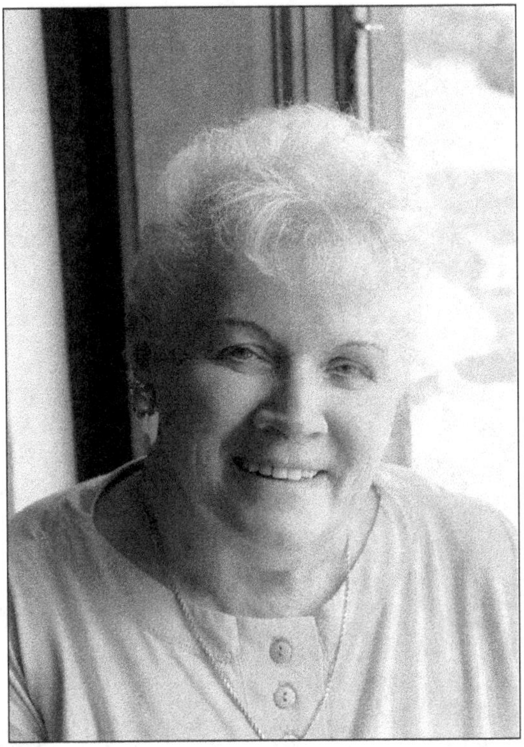

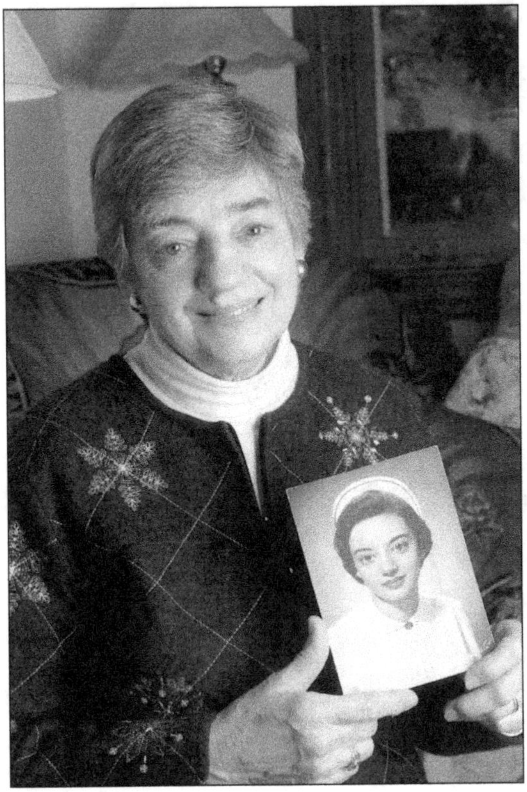

Constance Earle of Lombard, Illinois, was a 1955 graduate of St. Anne's School of Nursing. She remembers riding in floats and hearing the crowds cheer. She remembers the Brennan family, who attended the parade and held a sign to honor the St. Anne nurses. All the 13 Brennan children were born at St. Anne's Hospital. (Janet Boivin, "Chicago Nurses' Parade," *Nursing Spectrum*, January 2004; photo courtesy of *Nursing Spectrum*.)

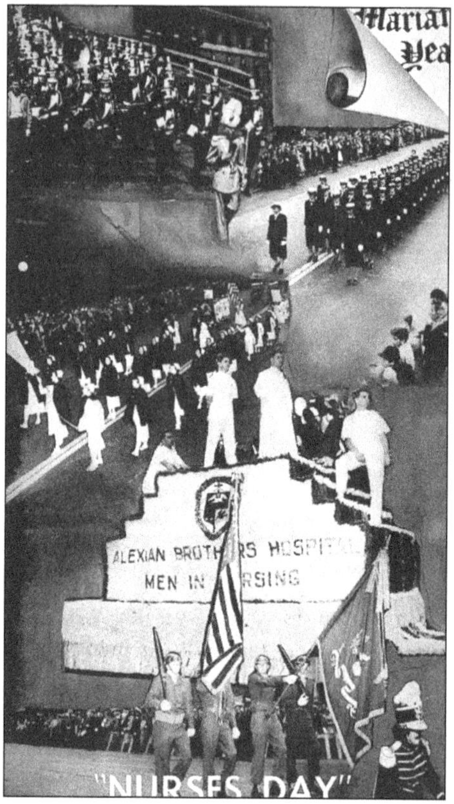
Marian Yea
ALEXIAN BROTH RS HOSPIT
MEN IN RSING
"NURSES DAY"

The *Novena Notes* cover of May 21, 1954, "pays tribute to Nurses Day. Under the sponsorship of the Sorrowful Mother Novena today, May 21, has been officially proclaimed Nurses Day throughout the state of Illinois. The climax of the celebration will be reached tonight during the giant parade and special Novena Service for nurses in the Novena National Shrine." (*Novena Notes*, May 21, 1954, 14.)

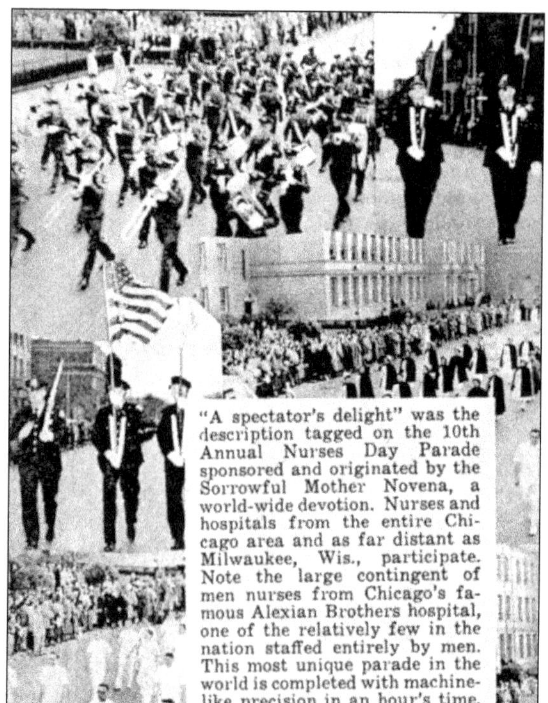
"A spectator's delight" was the description tagged on the 10th Annual Nurses Day Parade sponsored and originated by the Sorrowful Mother Novena, a world-wide devotion. Nurses and hospitals from the entire Chicago area and as far distant as Milwaukee, Wis., participate. Note the large contingent of men nurses from Chicago's famous Alexian Brothers hospital, one of the relatively few in the nation staffed entirely by men. This most unique parade in the world is completed with machine-like precision in an hour's time.

Marching bands certainly helped to make the Nurses Day Parade a spectator's delight. (*Novena Notes*, May 30, 1958, back cover.)

Bob Jaeger, R.N., was 19 years old when he was a student at Alexian Brothers Hospital School of Nursing. He marched in 1953, "We were all guys at Alexian Brothers and we did not mind marching in the parade if it gave us a chance to meet some young women." (Janet Boivin, *Nursing Spectrum*, January 2004; photo courtesy of *Nursing Spectrum*.)

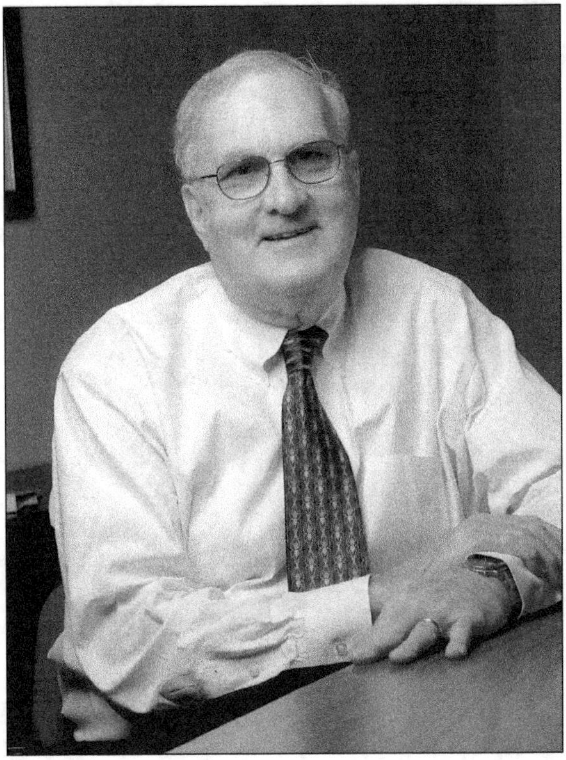

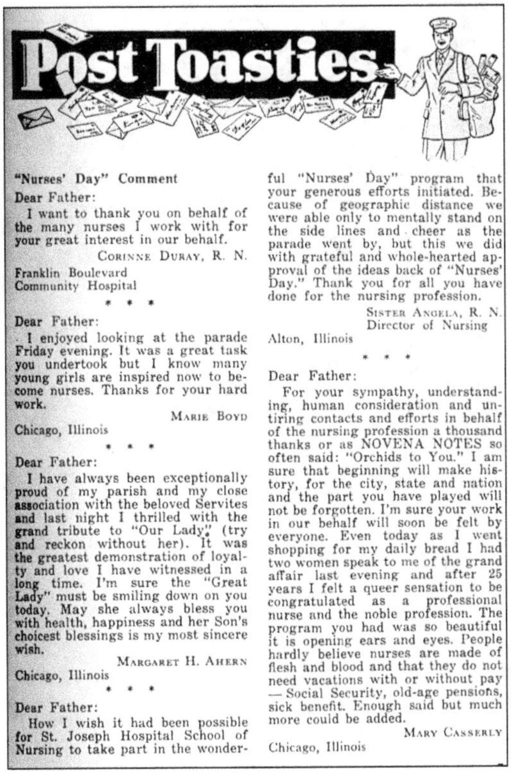

Post Toasties

"Nurses' Day" Comment

Dear Father:

I want to thank you on behalf of the many nurses I work with for your great interest in our behalf.

CORINNE DURAY, R. N.

Franklin Boulevard
Community Hospital

* * *

Dear Father:

I enjoyed looking at the parade Friday evening. It was a great task you undertook but I know many young girls are inspired now to become nurses. Thanks for your hard work.

MARIE BOYD

Chicago, Illinois

* * *

Dear Father:

I have always been exceptionally proud of my parish and my close association with the beloved Servites and last night I thrilled with the grand tribute to "Our Lady" (try and reckon without her). It was the greatest demonstration of loyalty and love I have witnessed in a long time. I'm sure the "Great Lady" must be smiling down on you today. May she always bless you with health, happiness and her Son's choicest blessings is my most sincere wish.

MARGARET H. AHERN

Chicago, Illinois

* * *

Dear Father:

How I wish it had been possible for St. Joseph Hospital School of Nursing to take part in the wonderful "Nurses' Day" program that your generous efforts initiated. Because of geographic distance we were able only to mentally stand on the side lines and cheer as the parade went by, but this we did with grateful and whole-hearted approval of the ideas back of "Nurses' Day." Thank you for all you have done for the nursing profession.

SISTER ANGELA, R. N.
Director of Nursing

Alton, Illinois

* * *

Dear Father:

For your sympathy, understanding, human consideration and untiring contacts and efforts in behalf of the nursing profession a thousand thanks or as NOVENA NOTES so often said: "Orchids to You." I am sure that beginning will make history, for the city, state and nation and the part you have played will not be forgotten. I'm sure your work in our behalf will soon be felt by everyone. Even today as I went shopping for my daily bread I had two women speak to me of the grand affair last evening and after 25 years I felt a queer sensation to be congratulated as a professional nurse and the noble profession. The program you had was so beautiful it is opening ears and eyes. People hardly believe nurses are made of flesh and blood and that they do not need vacations with or without pay — Social Security, old-age pensions, sick benefit. Enough said but much more could be added.

MARY CASSERLY

Chicago, Illinois

Notes of appreciation and gratitude from the nurses were published in the *Novena Notes*. Nurses wrote letters of thanks for having a Nurses Day Parade and expressed what the parade personally meant to them. (*Novena Notes*, Post Toasties, August 12, 1949, 7.)

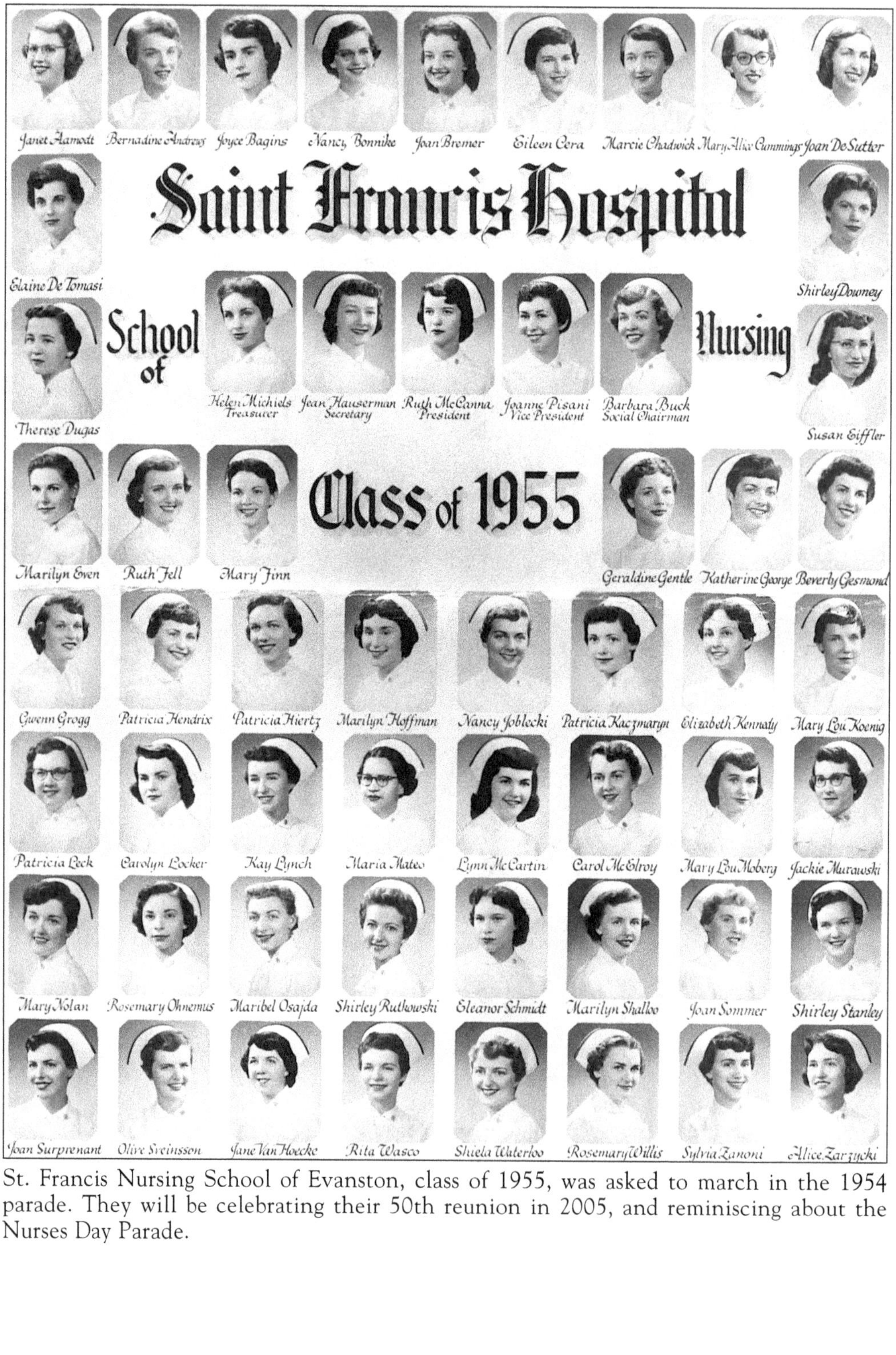

St. Francis Nursing School of Evanston, class of 1955, was asked to march in the 1954 parade. They will be celebrating their 50th reunion in 2005, and reminiscing about the Nurses Day Parade.

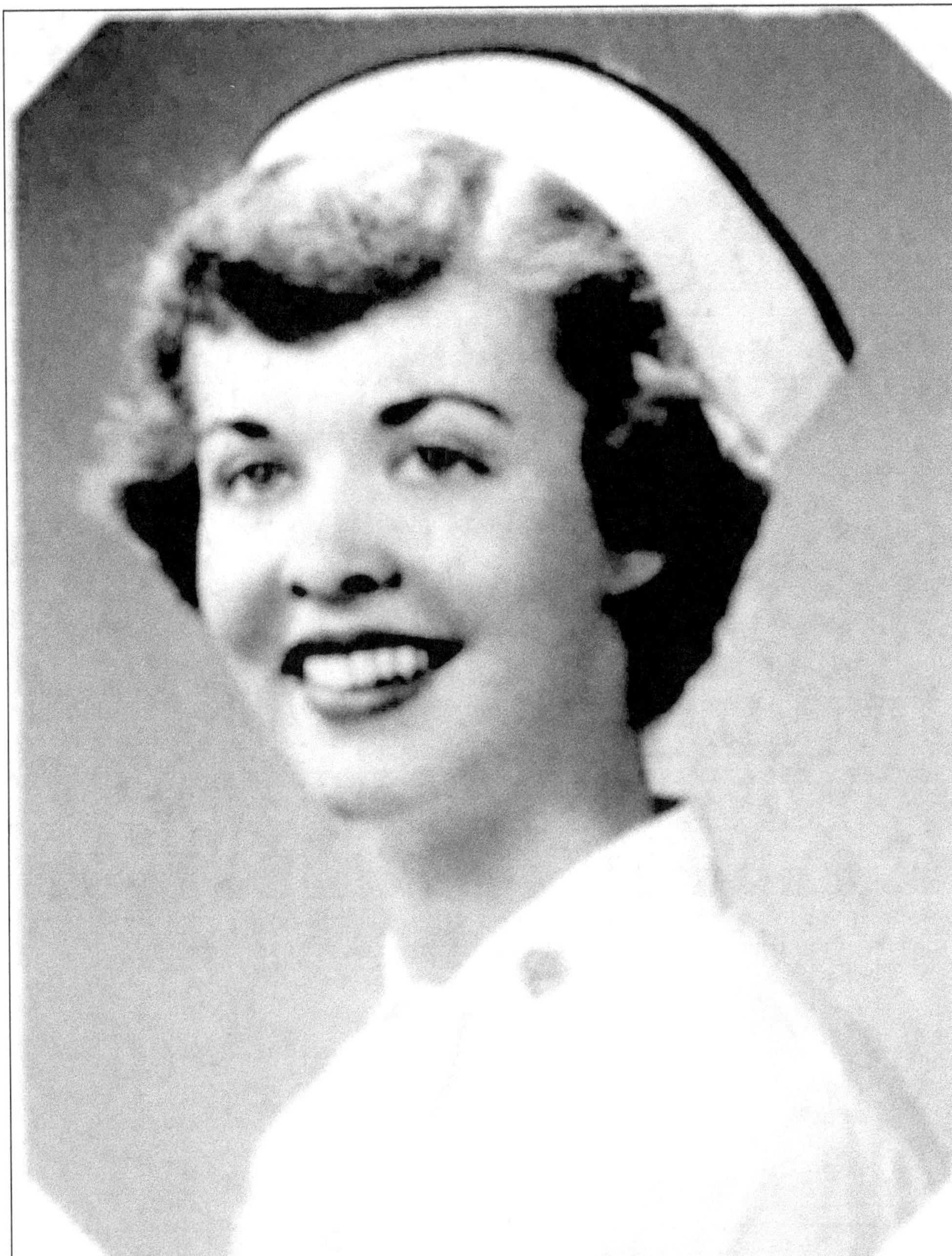

Barbara Buck

Barbara (nee Buck) Feltman, a 1955 St. Francis Hospital nursing graduate, remembers marching in the 1954 parade. Barbara remembers feeling proud to be a nurse and elegant in her grey nursing cape with red lining as she marched down Jackson Boulevard.

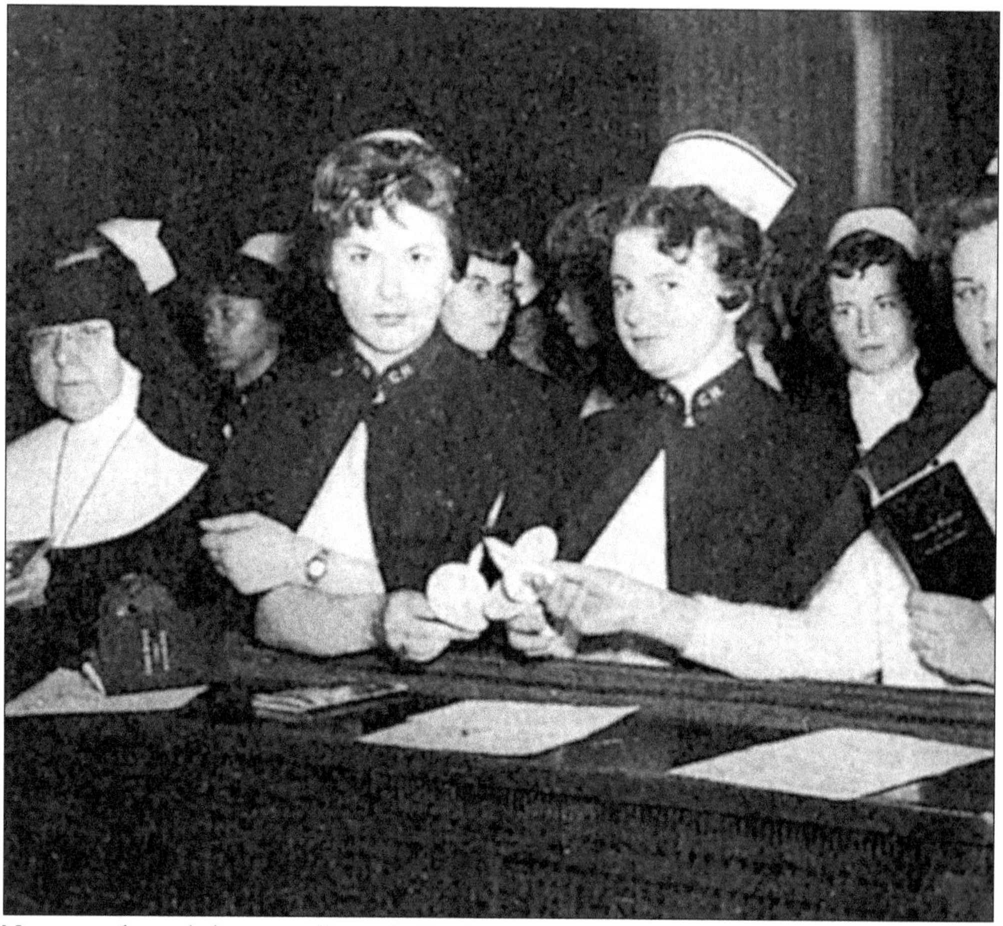

Nurses are shown lighting candles in the Basilica, preparing for the singing of the Lourdes Hymn at the end of the Benediction in 1958. This ceremony took place after the parade. (*Novena Notes*, May 30, 1958, 11.)

NATIONAL SHRINE
of the
SORROWFUL MOTHER NOVENA

Jackson Blvd. and Albany Ave., Chicago 12
NEvada 8-5800

HOURS OF NOVENA SERVICES

SHRINE — 7, 8, 9, 10 A.M., 3, 4, 5, 6, 7, 8, 9 P.M. UPPER CHURCH — 5:30 P.M.
Mass in Shrine at 6:30 A.M.
CONFESSIONS — Every Friday in rear of Shrine — 8 P.M. to 10 P.M.

NURSES' PLEDGE

(To be recited aloud by the nurses present at the special Sorrowful Mother Novena service at the Novena National Shrine on Nurses Day, 1956. The asterisks * signify pauses.)

I solemnly pledge myself before God and at this service of the Sorrowful Mother Novena* to pass my life in purity* and to practice my profession faithfully.*

I will abstain from whatever is deleterious and mischievous* and will not take or knowingly administer* any harmful drug.*

I will do all in my power to elevate the standard of my profession,* and will hold in confidence* all personal matters committed to my keeping,* and all family affairs coming to my knowledge* in the practice of my calling.*

With loyalty I will endeavor to aid the physician in his work* and devote myself to the welfare of those entrusted* to my care. So be it.*

Distinguished speaker for this Nurses Day special Novena service will be His Eminence Samuel Cardinal Stritch, Archbishop of Chicago

This is the nurses' pledge and invitation for nurses and supporters to attend the 1956 Novena service. (*Novena Notes*, May 18, 1956, 2.)

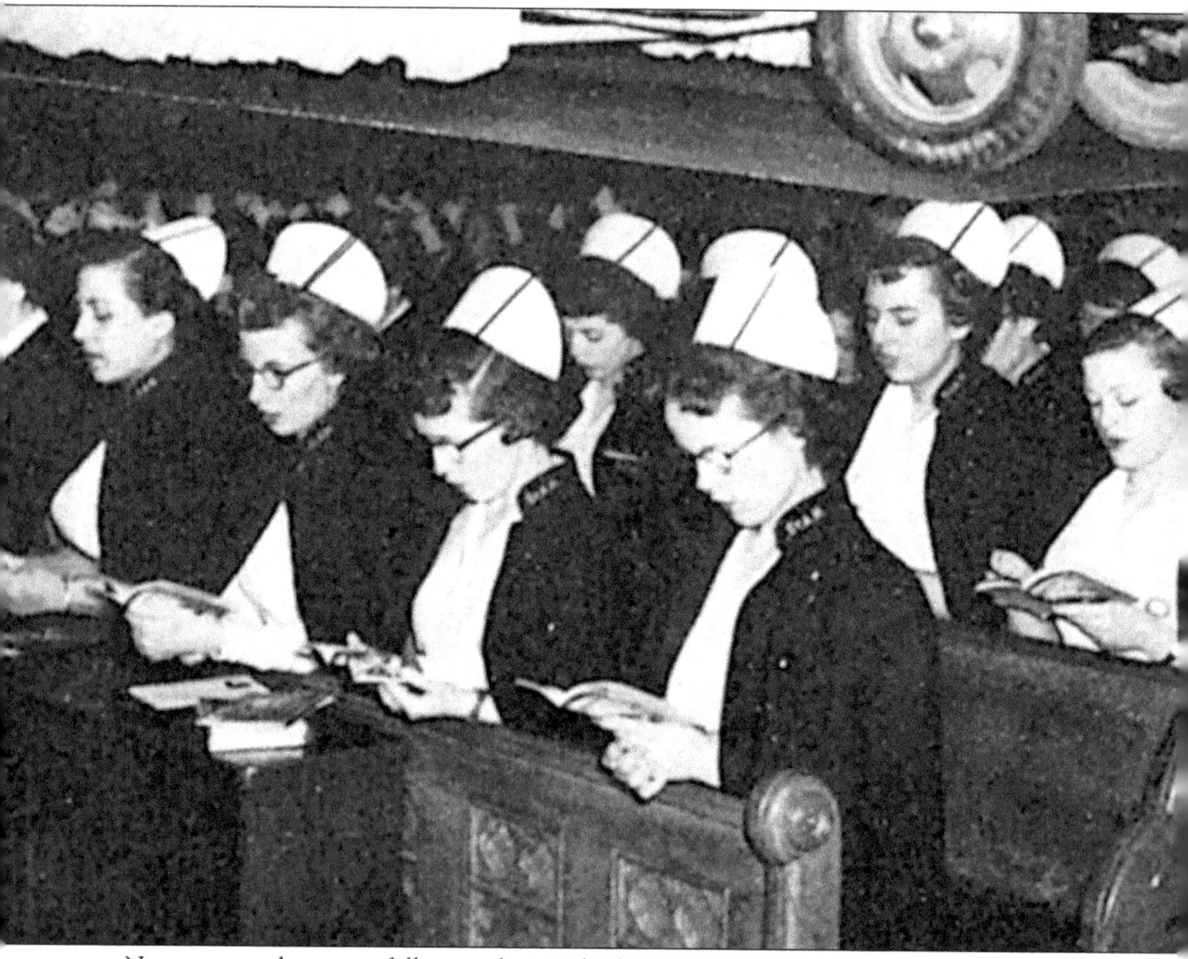

Nurses renew their vows following the parade. (*Novena Notes*, June 11, 1954, 12.)

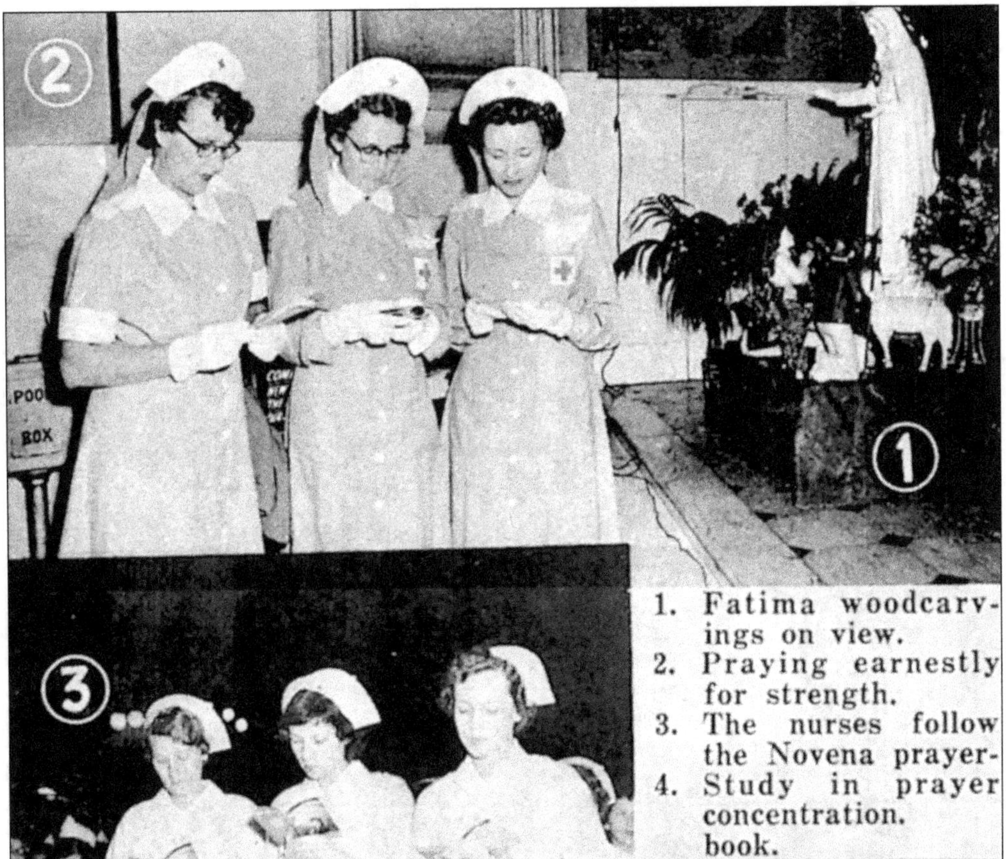

Nurses are seen here praying after the parade. (*Novena Notes*, October 6, 1950, 7.)

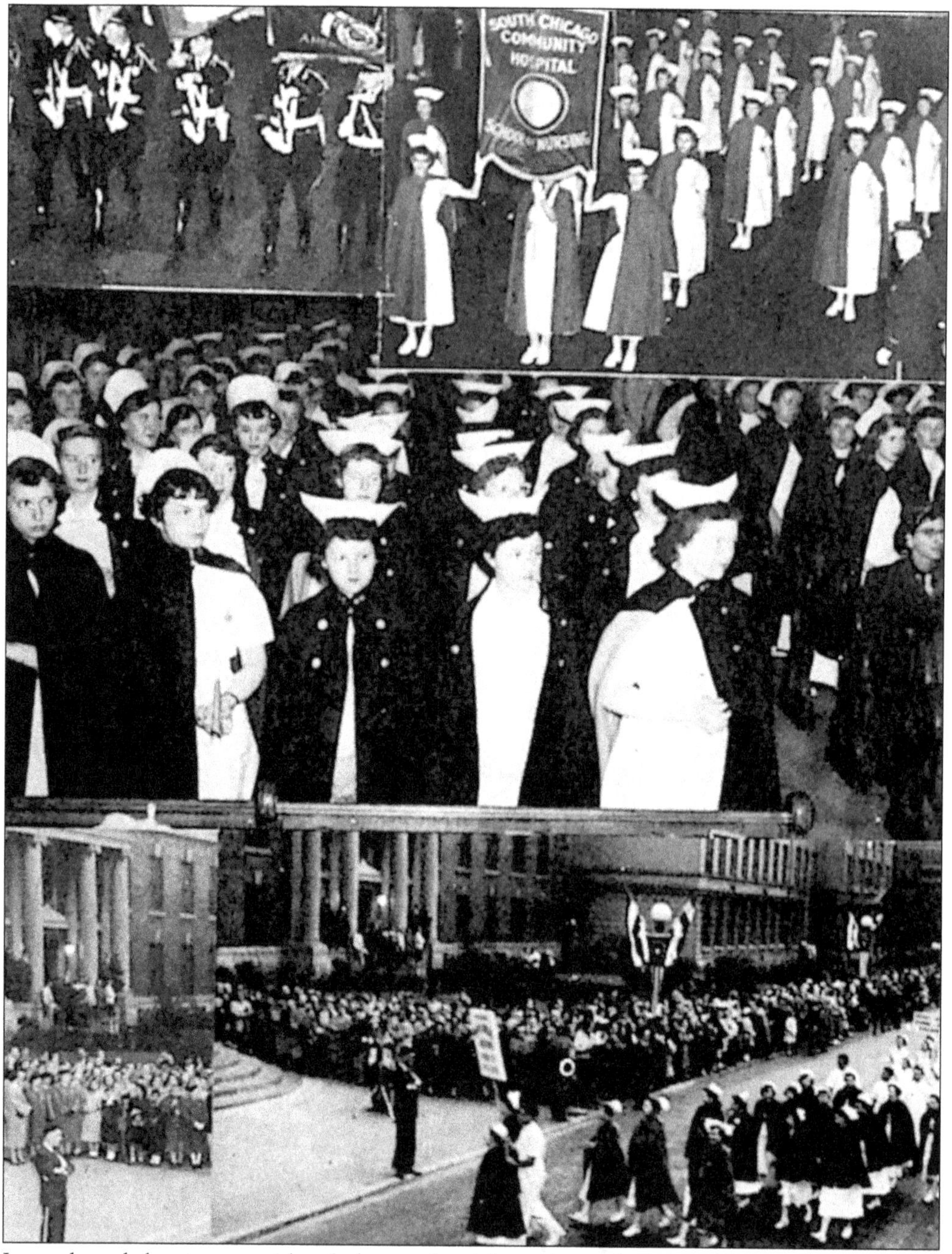

It was hoped that in nurses' lonely hours, the sight and sound of the 1954 parade would help them know that the public appreciated their vocation. (*Novena Notes*, June 11, 1954, 10.)

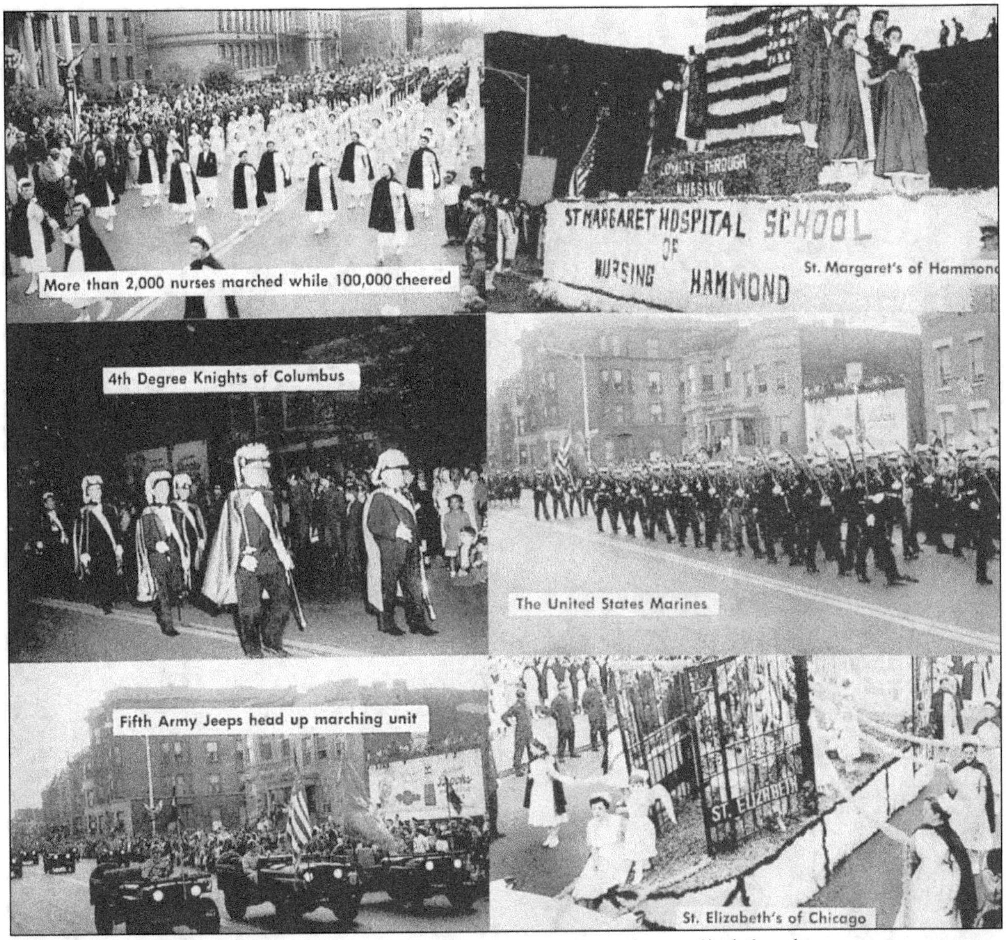
More than 2,000 nurses marched while 100,000 cheered
ST MARGARET HOSPITAL SCHOOL
OF
NURSING HAMMOND
St. Margaret's of Hammon
4th Degree Knights of Columbus
The United States Marines
Fifth Army Jeeps head up marching unit
ST. ELIZABETH
St. Elizabeth's of Chicago

While watching over bedsides or during trying moments that called for the utmost patience, memories of the Nurses Day Parade could provide comfort and inspiration to Chicago's nurses. (*Novena Notes*, June 8, 1956, 8–9.)

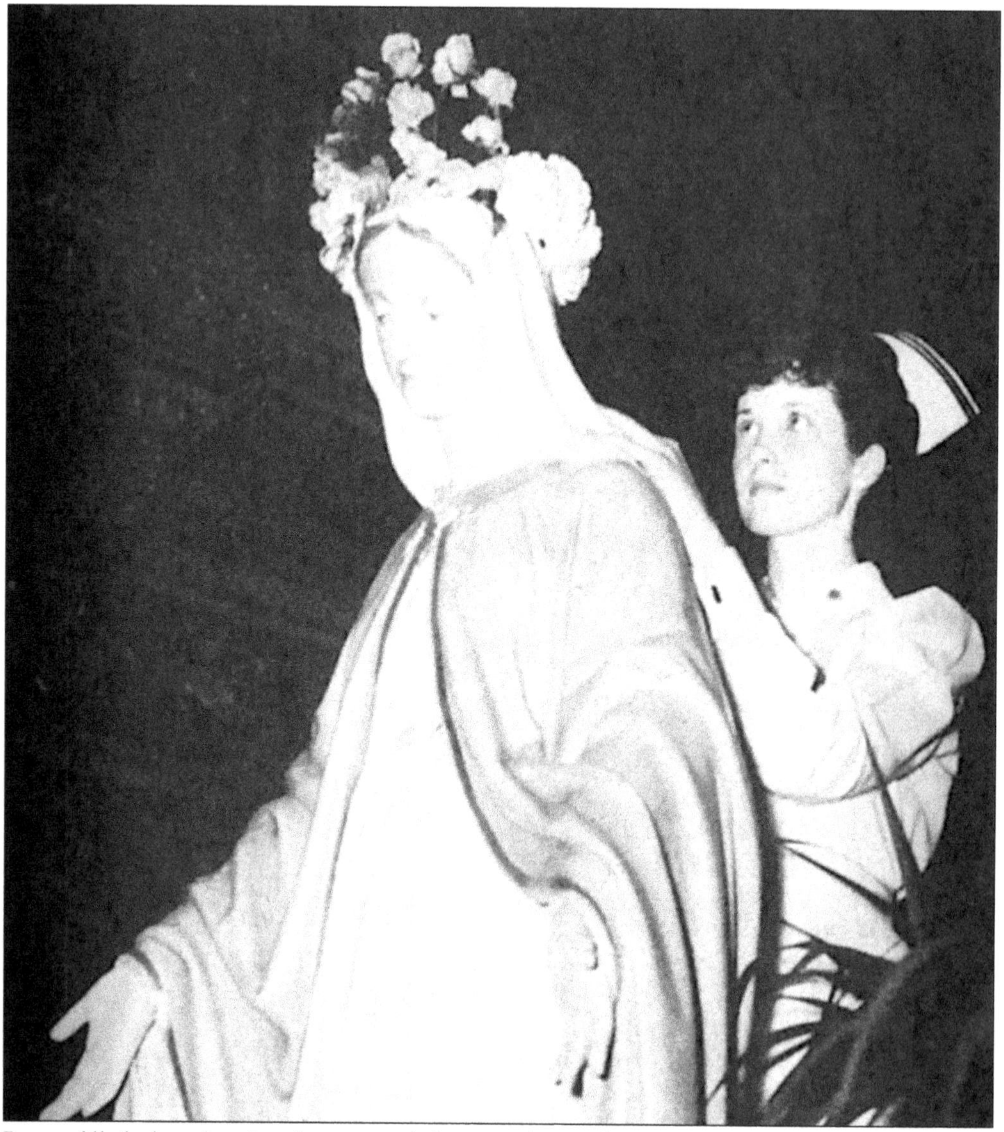

Roses filled the church after one of the parades to honor nurses. Roses are seen here decorating a statue of the Blessed Mother. (*Novena Notes*, June 11, 1954, 15.)

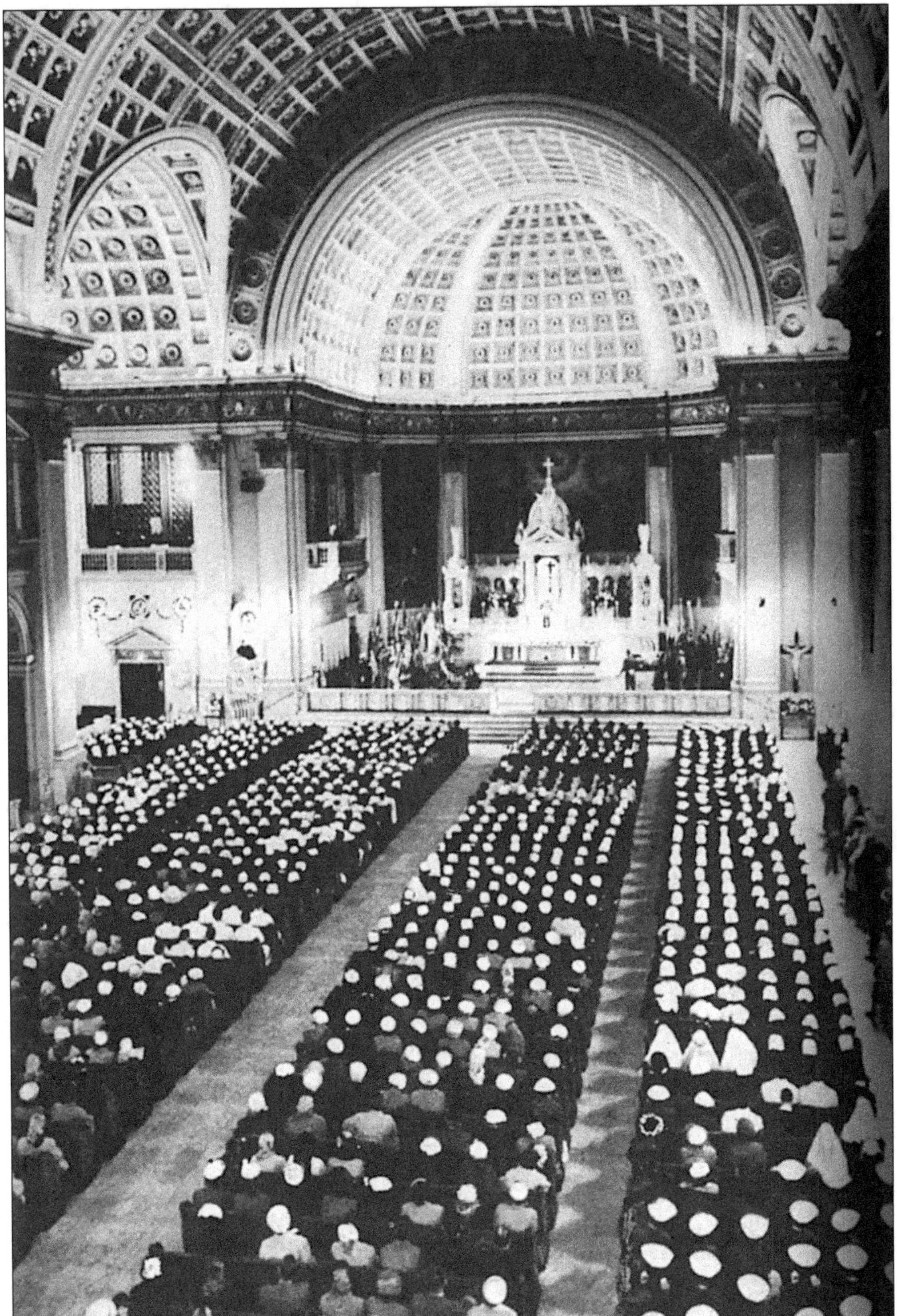

The parades were followed by a special Novena service in the National Shrine during which an inspiring discourse on the value of nursing was given. (*Novena Notes*, June 11, 1954, 16.)

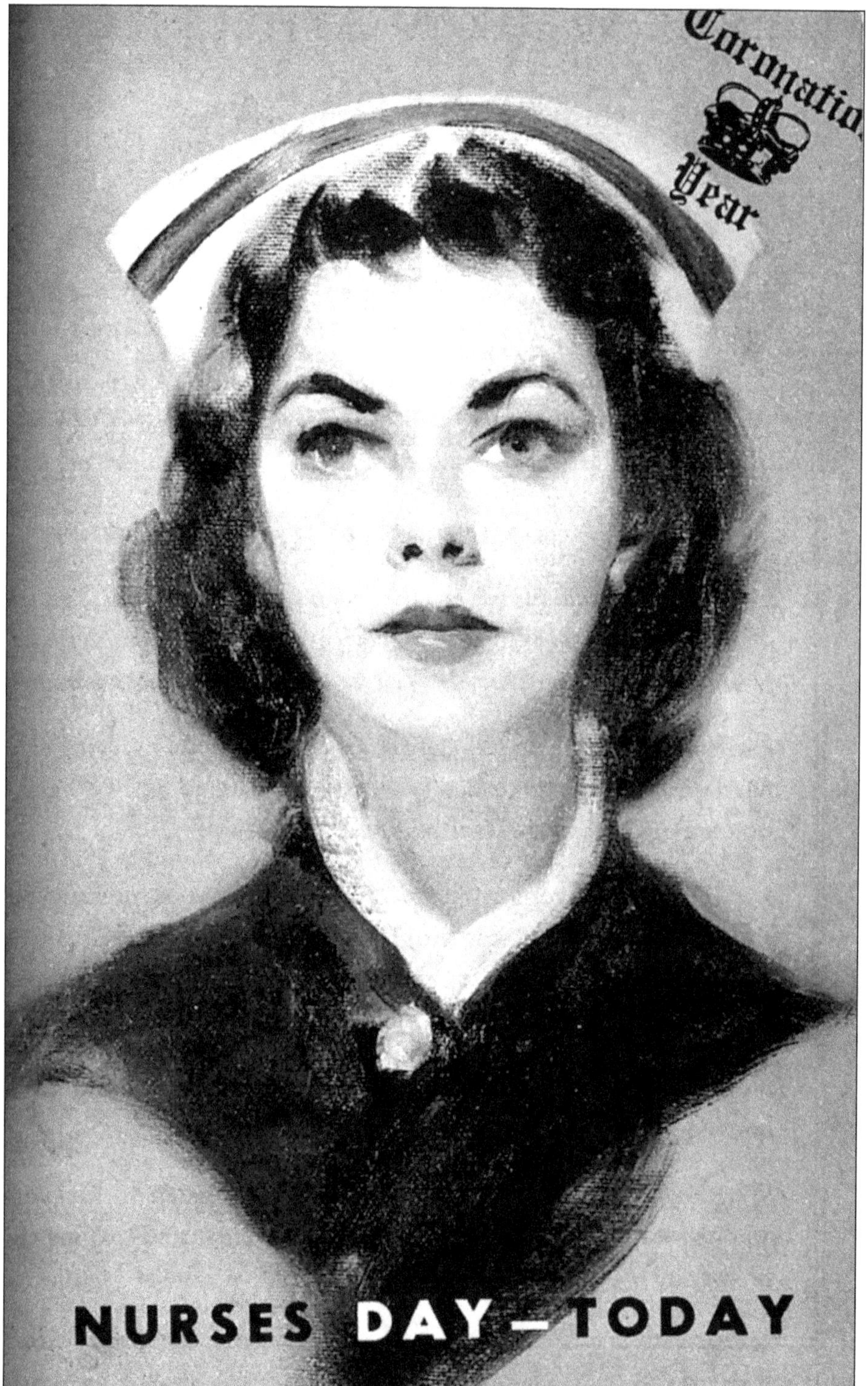

The cover of the *Novena Notes* of May 10, 1957, the night of the parade, salutes all nurses in the world. The artist was Richard Schmid whose murals grace the upper Basilica.

www.ingramcontent.com/pod-product-compliance
Lightning Source LLC
LaVergne TN
LVHW060412220926
848484LV00015B/2411